"There's a bit of Frank in all of us—broken yet hopeful, fallen yet getting back up, and often living our lives as smoldering sparks that never quite burn out, or ignite. To witness Frank's comeback story as he battles demons and comes to terms with failure, and to see him prevail and then soar provides inspiration at its absolute best."

—Mike Dooley, *New York Times* best-selling author of
Infinite Possibilities: The Art of Living Your Dreams

"Frank Ferrante has good news: Life's challenges aren't obstacles on our path to awakening—they are the path! Frank's honest, intimate sharing grounds us in the understanding that every aspect of what life presents is an opportunity to reconnect with our inherent integrity, authenticity, and joy."

—Michael Bernard Beckwith, author of *Life Visioning:
A Four-Stage Evolutionary Journey to Live as Divine Love*

"Frank's wit and his genuine, heartfelt wisdom make this book an inspiring journey of triumph—a true testimony to the human spirit's ability to rise against all adversity in the name of passion, love, and life. This is a must-read for anyone wanting to transform their body and live the life of their dreams."

—Jon Gabriel, international best-selling author and
creator of The Gabriel Method

"Frank Ferrante is the most unlikely of heroes. Through his outrageous, inspiring, and transparent adventures, we not only get to witness his transformation—we also get to witness and realize our own. Frank tells it like it is, brings us close, and makes us feel like family. It takes no time to fall in love with Frank. He speaks from the heart, showing he truly cares about us too."

—Jason Mraz

"People connect with Frank and see themselves, their story, their pains, their healing, their joys and their triumphs in what he shares with the world. Frank teaches what I know to be true about wellbeing—if you heal the heart you can heal the body."

—Dr. Michelle Robin, Your Wellness Connection founder and author of *Wellness on a Shoestring: Seven Habits for a Healthy Life*

May I Be
FRANK

May I Be FRANK

How I Changed My Ways,
Lost 100 Pounds, and Found Love

FRANK FERRANTE

North Atlantic Books
Berkeley, California

Published by
North Atlantic Books
P.O. Box 12327
Berkeley, California 94712

Cover photo by Cat Maida
Back cover photos by Cary Mosier and Gregg Marks
Cover design by Mary Ann Casler and Lisa Mia Ferrante
Book design by Mary Ann Casler
Printed in the United States of America

May I Be Frank: How I Changed My Ways, Lost 100 Pounds, and Found Love is sponsored and published by the Society for the Study of Native Arts and Sciences (dba North Atlantic Books), an educational nonprofit based in Berkeley, California, that collaborates with partners to develop cross-cultural perspectives, nurture holistic views of art, science, the humanities, and healing, and seed personal and global transformation by publishing work on the relationship of body, spirit, and nature.

North Atlantic Books' publications are available through most bookstores. For further information, visit our website at www.northatlanticbooks.com or call 800-733-3000.

Library of Congress Cataloging-in-Publication Data
Ferrante, Frank, 1951–
  May I be Frank : how I changed my ways, lost 100 pounds, and found love again / Frank Ferrante.
    pages cm
  ISBN 978-1-58394-879-8 — ISBN 978-1-58394-880-4
1. Ferrante, Frank, 1951- 2. Ferrante, Frank, 1951—Health. 3. Ferrante, Frank, 1951—In motion pictures. 4. Overweight persons—United States—Biography. 5. Drug addicts—United States—Biography. 6. Weight loss—United States. 7. Drug addiction—Treatment--United States. 8. Holistic medicine—United States. 9. Self-actualization (Psychology)—United States. 10. Documentary films—United States. I. Title.
CT275.F4826A3 2015
155.2—dc23   2014030367

1 2 3 4 5 6 7 8 VERSA 20 19 18 17 16 15

Printed on recycled paper

To my beautiful children, Lisa Mia Ferrante and Nicholas Frank Ferrante.
And to Cat Maida, who effortlessly shows me what love looks like every day.
I could never have done this without you. Thank you for choosing me.

Table of Contents

Foreword

I knew I liked Frank the minute I met him; he seemed to be "clear," whatever that means. I didn't feel baggage, projection, or walls of any kind. He just seemed vulnerable and strong and kind.

In today's world, just being "vulnerable and strong and kind" is the mark of someone who has done whatever it takes to become that way. Sad statement about the times we live in, but true.

I had no idea then what he had been through in his life, what his struggles or challenges or triumphs had been. I had no idea he'd lost a gazillion pounds, or had starred in a documentary, or was a cult figure of sorts due to both those things. But I did feel he had a profound knowing of some kind. I had a sense that absolutely nothing got past him.

Reading Frank's book, I came to understand his journey from lost-in-the-dark to found-in-the-light. I'm excited that others will find hope in his journey that inspires them along their own. Just as a picture is worth a thousand words, the true story of one person's transformation is worth a thousand treatises on what breaks a human being and what makes them heal. Frank has been broken in his life, and Frank has healed. Just reading his story gives the reader inspiration with which to more fully live theirs.

Frank has only just begun to share with the world the gifts he has received from doing his work, opening his heart, and changing his mind. This book is a personal testament to the power of God, and also to the power of Frank ... for humbly presenting himself before the Creator of the Universe and taking step after step toward redemption and hope.

What Frank has received, he is ready to give. And what he has seen, he shows all of us who are willing to see. Reader, get ready: Frank's about to touch your heart.

Marianne Williamson
Los Angeles
October, 2014

1

Sign from the Universe

My New Age friends inspired by spiritual leanings remind me to be present to the "signs" offered up by the Universe. I politely nod in agreement as my mind churns out disclaimers: *Yeah, right! What the hell is the "Universe" anyway besides trillions of stars? Send me a memo when you find out.* Even though I voluntarily took up residence in San Francisco, I harbored deep skepticism about all this California dreaming.

Why would a blue-collar Sicilian guy from Brooklyn live in San Francisco, of all places? The reason was professional—in 2005 I was accepted into the humanities graduate program at San Francisco State, an achievement of particular importance since I waited until the age of fifty to get a high school diploma. I should have gotten it sooner, but I was "busy."

One day I received a call from my cousin Michelangelo (yes, that's his real name, and no, he's not a ninja turtle) who told me he was ill and out of sorts. Before going to see him, I drove to Le Video, a video store specializing in foreign films located in the Inner Sunset near the intersection of 9th Street and Irving in San Francisco. I thought I'd rent some Italian movies—cheerful neorealism, perhaps—and watch them with my cousin.

In the distance I saw "a sign." Rather than a metaphor, the Universe, in its infinite wisdom, sent me a sign I could easily comprehend: a well-lit billboard over a restaurant that read "Café Gratitude."

Gratitude is a central virtue in the 12 Step world; I assumed someone from AA was being cute and clever with the name for a coffee shop. I walked toward this Café Gratitude anticipating a clientele of recovering addicts and alcoholics. I was about to tumble down a rabbit hole that would change the direction of my life—it was one of those moments when going left instead of right would have altered me forever.

It was a gloomy February night in San Francisco. The sidewalks and streets glistened from the dampness. The fog hung in the air like a dreary gray curtain. The atmosphere reflected my dismal internal landscape. I was reaping the rewards of my many years of hard living—weighing three hundred pounds and feeling unimaginably lonely. So lonely in fact, I sometimes rang my own doorbell to hear what a visitor would sound like. My relationships were toxic because I was toxic. I felt lost and disconnected from everything. I was filled with self-loathing. I felt like I was dying.

I stood in front of the café and peered through the large storefront window. The place was warmly lit with only a few people inside. Hemingway's "A Well-Lighted Place" came to mind. Standing on the other side of a large front window, a pretty young woman with an olive complexion and two long auburn braids—she looked like Pocahontas—smiled brightly and innocently as if to say, "It is okay, you can come in. It's safe here." For a moment, she reminded me of my daughter.

I sucked in my gut and opened the door, jangling a little bell. I was met with a barrage of hearty salutations from the young staff. "Hi! Welcome! C'mon in! Glad you're here!" For a lonely guy like me it was like hearing eighteen years of greetings in ten seconds. I walked up to a smiling twenty-something hipster, shook hands with him, and said, "Hey man, I had to get a cup of coffee at Café Gratitude. I figure somebody here is in recovery." He looked back at me and said, "We're all recovering from something . . . aren't we?"

I immediately knew he wasn't in recovery and assumed he had just smoked a joint before coming to work. As I looked around, I noticed the absence of an espresso machine. *What, no coffee in this place? Not to mention no recovering boozers or dope fiends.* There wasn't even a stove. It didn't look like any restaurant I had ever seen or would have normally entered. Ryland, my twenty-something waiter and host, noticed the perplexed look on my face. "We're a raw food, vegan restaurant," he explained. "We just opened a few months ago."

My first thought was, *Raw food! How do you cook that?* Up until that time, I thought vegan was a planet. I was convinced that humans were born to eat cooked meat; I was also deeply committed to raspberry white truffle cheesecake and fried chicken—a dietary relationship which announced itself through my waistline.

Despite my confusion about the menu (I couldn't decipher the entrée items as each went by an affirmation such as the "I Am Healthy" green juice), the café was a radiant wonderland filled with happy, shiny-looking young people. I am by nature an extrovert who can be comfortable in most situations—if I'm not depressed or bored. I was also a hippie in my youth. Yet around this crowd I felt like a cross between Richard Nixon and Don Rickles. "This isn't just a restaurant. It's a school of transformation," said Ryland. And I found myself thinking, *This really nice kid is in his hippie phase of life. I don't buy anything he's saying, but it's a refreshing perspective.*

Even though I was fat enough to cause an eclipse of the sun, I felt unseen. But these young New Age types made me feel comfortable, wanted, and visible. I felt a kindness and a sincere welcoming spirit here. So I started frequenting the place. It certainly wasn't about the food. I may have eaten a salad or two of sprouts, after which I'd march out to find the nearest Indian buffet and gorge myself—I needed more than leaves to get around, or so I thought.

Another part of my being needed nurturing just as much as my body. These bright, shiny young idealists were stirring it. My soul was crying out for connection, and my heart was yearning for love. That first night, unbeknownst to me, I found both.

To generate meaningful conversation, the staff at Café Gratitude pose to customers a "Question of the Day." When Ryland asked me, "What do you want to do before you die?" I responded without hesitation: "I want to fall in love one more time, but I don't think anyone will love me with

3

this body." Ryland leaned closer. "Frankie, want to do something about it? Would you like to be part of an experiment?"

That word "experiment" captured my full attention. *What do you want me to be? A guinea pig? I guess we're all guinea pigs in our own life experiments anyway, so what the hell!*

"Let us become your transformational cheerleaders?"

"What do you mean?" I was both intrigued and suspicious. *Are they cheerleaders for a cult group, and am I being recruited?*

"You come in here, and you eat this food," he said, " and you allow us to be your transformational cheerleaders so that you can shed whatever you're carrying: the shame, the weight, the discontent, and really love yourself so that someone else can love you. And we'll film everything."

I was getting high counsel and an offer of help from an idealistic twenty-year-old. I was old enough to be his father, but I was already surrounded by twenty-something students in graduate school, so some kind of co-generational karma was already at work in my life. Psychologists claim that practicing addicts are in a state of arrested development, and that their emotional growth stagnates at the age they become addicts. Maybe I was staring my own emotional timeline in the face.

Ryland later confessed that he saw me as this fat, sometimes obnoxious Italian from Brooklyn who can be endearing when I want to be. Maybe he thought I was a challenge, a project worth undertaking, and not as hopeless as I thought I was. *What do I have to lose except maybe some weight?*

Besides the weight problem, I suffered from a slew of issues, my legacy as an ex-junkie and alcoholic: hepatitis C, chronic fatigue, joint pain, severe depression, and a libido that was all but a distant memory. I was taking a daily fistful of prescribed meds to help me feel better. Instead, I felt like death warmed-over, I was afraid I might live. Like millions of people, I had issues. Mine brought me eye to eye with the Angel of Death.

At that time, I was an unemployed, full-time student working on my master's in humanities. I struggled to keep pace with the youngsters who surrounded me in class. Grants or student loans were my source of income. I frequently woke up with the Four Horsemen of the Apocalypse

4

trampling the inside of my head. At fifty-four years old, I felt like the least likely candidate for a major personal transformation.

"Okay, I'll do it," I blurted, even though I was thinking, *What is this going to cost me? I don't have a clue what I am agreeing to, but I don't think it will hurt me. If I don't like what comes up, I can always get in the wind.*

There is no logic as to why I verbally agreed to something so open-ended, except that I had quickly grown to trust this young man. I figured I'd drink some wheatgrass, eat some nuclear-powered rabbit food, lose some weight, and then move on.

Little did I know. . . .

2

Into the Rabbit Hole, Week One

W e met so I could sign over my life and my free will to Ryland and his two equally young fellow conspirators and restaurant coworkers, Cary and Conor. By a stroke of cosmic poetic timing, the following ceremony took place on Valentine's Day, the day dedicated to love and romance, experiences I thought would remain in my past.

We sat at a table in Café Gratitude, the three amigos and me, looking over a contract they had drawn up that defined my actions and behaviors for the next six weeks. As I recited the list out loud, my stomach began to churn in apprehension.

"I agree to eat three meals at Café Gratitude, which are approved by either Matthew or Terces." (They're the owners of Café Gratitude.)

"I agree to complete my daily logbook every day, all portions, at breakfast." *Sounds like one of my school assignments.*

"I agree to do my daily affirmations every day when I wake up and every day before I go to bed." *I don't know about this one.*

"I agree to walk fifteen minutes every day." *I can do that.*

"I agree to order my food in its affirmation name." (Remember that all of the restaurant's menu items are identified by a short affirmation phrase.)

"I agree to drink a gallon of water a day." *So goodbye to sleeping through the night without interruption.*

"I agree to call either Cary, Conor, or Ryland and communicate whether I have completed my daily agreement." I rolled my eyes at this one, but deep down, I was glad to be connecting with someone at this level.

"I agree to be on time for all my appointments." *I think I can do that.*

"I agree to not degrade myself." *That will be a tough one.*

"I agree to relate to my food as my medicine and my medicine as my food." *What the hell does that mean?*

"I agree to be coachable and be in this project with a beginner's mind." *I will do my best.*

"I understand and agree to relate to Cary, Conor, and Ryland as my coaches in the transformation in my life."

"Wait a minute," I balked, feeling a welling up of resistance. "What does that mean?"

Conor spoke up, "We are your coaches. Like, if you're an athlete and the game that we're playing is the transformation of your life. You're the player in that, and we're the coach. And we just like you to know that, when we say things to you, it's because we are coaching you in surrendering."

"Okay," I said, making a trial run of surrender. "I agree." But my thoughts were riffing along the lines of, *Holy shit! These guys are serious. Wait a minute, what do they really have in mind; what am I really getting myself into?* I immediately began seeking out loopholes. Most addicts would make excellent lawyers—if a loophole exists, an addict will find it.

I signed the contract, and, one by one, each of the three signed their names below my signature. The agreement was rooted in integrity and not enforceable. That alarmed me because that gave the document a deepening gravitas. I began to feel a low murmur of anxiety within.

The three amigos also confessed they'd been thinking about finding an unhealthy fat guy, filming him on a raw food diet, and making a film the opposite of *Super Size Me*, the 2004 documentary about a man who lived on a thirty-day diet of fast food. When they first talked about documenting our little experiment, I didn't know what it meant to be filmed. I had visions of young kids with the 2005 equivalent of an 8-mm movie camera.

I thought it might be like a school project or something for Myspace, which is to say that I didn't take the idea too seriously. None of them had any film experience or even owned a movie camera. I had the most film experience because I had seen the most movies.

Young enough to be my sons, these three handsome hipsters/coaches/cheerleaders were short-haired, clean-shaven, and clean-cut Boy Scout types, just like the three sons in the ancient television series, but definitely didn't think like or embody mainstream characters. Their attire consisted of colorful hippie T-shirts, eclectic headgear, and skinny jeans. All three were committed to a spiritual path and personal transformation. Cary, Conor, and Ryland were so young they could have shared the same razor for six months and it still would've remained sharp. Together they interacted as the ingredients of a tossed salad. I could separate them and like each kid on his own, but in the end they were from one big bowl of lovable lunacy.

Ryland Engelhart, a son of the Café Gratitude owners, was effervescent. He was like a squirrel on meth. In a good way. He had a childlike wonderment and a wide-eyed innocence about him and exuded positive enthusiasm in everything he did. Forgetful because he was always in the moment, he sometimes seemed a little eccentric.

Ryland's half-brother was Cary Mosier, a sort of brooding existentialist, deeply contemplative, and by far the most serious of the three. He seemed the hardest to read, darkest of the three, and more shadowy. He had an acute business sense, was a talented photographer, and was always trying something new like playing the guitar or drums. Cary was a technologically savvy, no-nonsense sort of guy.

Their childhood friend, Conor Gaffney, was more grounded and mature for his age, very kind, thoughtful, and happy. If my daughter brought him home, I would instantly be okay with him, which is quite a statement from a protective Sicilian father. Conor played bass for the easy-going, Woodstock-infused "Makepeace Brothers" rock band that had once toured with Jason Mraz. At the time I had absolutely no clue who Jason Mraz was.

I found it interesting that Cary, Conor, and Ryland were completely different people but operating with a similar lifestyle paradigm. Put the three kids together and our interactions felt playful, like I was the older, wounded boomer lion and they were the mid-sized millennial cubs. I felt comfortable with them, as if we were an instant family.

After signing the contract I felt a murmuring suspicion that I just joined a cause I didn't fully understand and might end up regretting. On the other hand, I felt a cautious optimism: *Who knows? This could be something great.*

Irrespective of my doubts, I was desperate enough to do just about anything to generate a shift in my life. My internal world had become a film noir, the colors were drying, and my world was shrinking. Three New Age vegans—what harm could they possibly do? So I took a chance on them and on myself. I wasn't worried that I'd be drinking the Kool-Aid in some suicide ritual, but if there was even a hint of cult-like tendencies, I would initiate a fast and furious exit.

Like Throwing Up Verbiage

The next morning I went back to the restaurant to drink their version of Kool-Aid, wheatgrass "medicine." Thus began my daily regimen. This first week was a strictly liquid diet: four ounces of wheatgrass, three times a day, chased down by a smoothie. The mere thought of going without solid food for a week evoked that scene from *Apocalypse Now* in which Marlon Brando is rasping "the horror." I would try not to let that feeling spoil my appetite for resolution.

My introduction to this brave new world of nutrition came courtesy of Matthew Engelhart, the aforementioned co-owner of Café Gratitude and one of its guiding-light gurus. He's a thin guy around my age with graying hair and wire-rimmed glasses. He looks a lot like his son Ryland. Under the brim of his blue baseball cap Matthew was usually smiling, which struck me as both disarming and suspicious. We sat on the café's outdoor patio to test whether I could handle my first shot of wheatgrass juice without gagging uncontrollably and throwing up.

Wheatgrass looked like the bright green slush left behind in the lawnmower bag after cutting a damp yard. Matthew and Ryland proceeded to tell me that almost every nutrient on the planet can be found in the stuff, particularly chlorophyll, and I'd be drinking four ounces of it at a time, three times a day. Oh, lucky me!

"The taste is repulsive to the degree you need to detox," Matthew noted, as I eyed the stuff, sniffed it, and tried to control my gag reflex.

"Oh, how convenient," I replied.

"Medicine, remember, it's medicine," Matthew tried to reassure me.

I dropped my head back and gulped it down as fast as I could, just like a shot of vodka or tequila. Oh, man, talk about God-awful tasting. It was everything I feared and more.

Ryland reminded me that my habit of drinking four or five shots of espresso every day had failed to keep my energy up, but he assured me that wheatgrass would be a more natural and healthy substitute. "Right," I confessed. "I'm just using coffee like an amphetamine."

I had noticed that Matthew's energy level, along with that of his wife Terces, remained consistent from 9:00 in the morning to 9:00 at night—not up, not down. Overall wellness at their age was attractive to me. If consuming stuff from the back of a lawnmower was the answer to all my problems, maybe I needed to give this medicine a chance.

After the wheatgrass juice, they had me drink a smoothie made of coconut milk, figs, cacao, and a bunch of other healthy stuff. That tasted much, much better. Of course, after wheatgrass, motor oil would have tasted good to me. "No caffeine after today," Matthew instructed. "If you get headaches, have a little bit of black tea, but wean yourself off that, too."

"This is going to change your life," interjected Ryland. *Going to change my life? Sounds like an evangelist seeking a convert.*

By the second day, I realized the tremendous weight of what I had signed up for. I surrounded myself with these smiling and warm people so that they would reflect back to me my integrity, my word of honor, and they expected me to follow through. I started to get a little worried. *Oh, shit, how am I going to do this? How can I survive on three small liquid meals a day, one drink of which is so horrible that it gags me at every gulp and makes me want to puke?*

I nevertheless felt compelled to hold up my end of the bargain, though I had serious doubts about meeting the challenge. My feeling of trepidation was compounded by the daily affirmations they insisted I recite in order to build up my self-esteem. They didn't want me to demean myself anymore, yet the verbiage they instructed me to regurgitate made me feel like a phony.

Matthew: "So you just repeat after me, okay? . . . I, Frank,"

Me: "I, Frank,"

Matthew: "do love me,"

Me: "do love me,"

Matthew: "my body's vigor"

Me: "my body's vigor"

Matthew: "and harmony."

Me: "and harmony."

Matthew: "I am"

Me: "I am"

Matthew: "perfect health,"

Me: "perfect health,"

Matthew: "radiant beauty,"

Me: "raaaaaaadiant beauty," *Let's switch this up for variety's sake*, I am thinking, though what I am really doing is trying to use humor to distance myself from what I am feeling.

Matthew: "and divine energy."

Me: "and divine energy."

Matthew: "I now hold in my mind"

Me: "I now hold in my mind"

Matthew: "this new image of myself"

Me: "this new image of myself"

Matthew: "as a thriving,"

Me: "as a thriving,"

Matthew: "flourishing,"

Me: "flourishing,"

Matthew: "and gloriously beautiful person."

Me: "and gloriously beautiful person."

At the conclusion, every muscle in my body felt ready to split in half. I couldn't get past the conviction that affirmations were a form of denial and magical thinking. I felt disingenuous and unnatural, as if a lie of this magnitude would provoke God himself to dish out a proper retribution.

Each morning following a glass of freshly mowed wheatgrass, I looked myself in the mirror and almost burst a blood vessel by mid-sentence of "I, Frank, do love me, my body's vigor and harmony. I am in perfect health, radiant beauty, and divine energy." For years attack thoughts had echoed in my head. I felt ashamed and embarrassed about challenging the old beliefs about myself. When I began these affirmations, which were so sacrosanct to Café Gratitude management (remember that their menu was created around them—would you really care for an "I Am Awesome" smoothie?), I questioned the ability of my mind to magnetically attract anything other than food, negative thoughts, or psycho-pharmaceuticals.

The idea that your mind can heal your body or manifest change through creative and positive visualizations isn't a modern concept drawn from that New Age movie *The Secret*. Instead, it draws its sources from ancient Eastern mysticism, of which credibility had been obliterated in our part of the world upon the Industrial Revolution when a scientific and materialistic world view got a vice grip on our Western minds. It then took a while to come around to the idea that science and metaphysics are connected, or that spirituality and psychology seamlessly overlap in distinctive ways.

I completed the affirmation ritual anyway; I did it because it felt like I didn't have anything to lose and I had given my word, which was the last shred of self-respect that stood between my survival and the dark precipice of extinction.

On day two of this experiment I made it in to Café Gratitude for "breakfast," but I couldn't rally myself to make it in for lunch. I phoned my coaches and told them, "I'm shivering, and I've got the runs." I don't think they completely believed me because Ryland came over to check on my condition. "It's just the detox," Ryland tried to reassure me. "All that wheatgrass in your system is probably just sucking all the toxins out of your body."

I wanted to trust Ryland, but my body was telling me to get the fuck back to New York. *God knows what's really in that grass. Maybe it's New Age Kool-Aid after all, and I'm slowly being poisoned. Or worse, it's all bullshit.*

New Age Storm Troopers in My Kitchen

The idea of consuming wheatgrass juice and raw foods and abstaining from wheat, sugar, dairy, and coffee soon began to freak me out. And I had forty days to go! My obsessive thoughts around the rituals of eating began to haunt me: I counted on rich, tasty food for pleasure and for distraction from personal woes.

Even though I knew my coaches would eventually be coming to inspect my pantry, it was a little unnerving when they stormed up three flights of stairs and burst into my small apartment flaunting trash bags. I was studying for a graduate school assignment when they took me completely by surprise. (Having each been given a key to my humble abode, they, I guessed, wanted to periodically check on me to reassure themselves that I had not committed hari-kari or otherwise flaked out on them.)

They went straight for my refrigerator and, after opening up two of the huge plastic trash bags, began emptying the contents with the disapproving glee of inspectors from the New Age Food and Drug Administration. "This is going to change your life," Cary declared. Ryland pulled a bag of frozen peas from the freezer and dangled it contemptuously. "Come on, Frank. These have got to go. Maybe they're raw, but they're frozen, and they've got no nutrition."

"Okay, okay," I replied as the frozen peas landed with a splat in the bottom of a trash bag.

"Look, he's got fried chicken!" Ryland exclaimed, pulling out a plate covered with cellophane. "A double no-no. Fried and chicken. That will go right to your belly."

"I haven't eaten any of that crap," I responded with mock horror.

"Yeah, right," replied Cary.

"The mother lode! Jackpot!" Conor yelped, holding up one of my favorite cuts of steak, a T-bone.

"Rancher's Reserve. Yum," Ryland chimed in with an edge of sarcasm. They continued pulling old chicken nuggets, cheese, butter, pasta, sugar, salt, and most everything else from my refrigerator and cabinets and trashing them. I couldn't bear to watch anymore and turned away to distract myself. "He can't even be with this. He left the room now," Conor said, punctuated with a laugh.

Within just a few minutes my kitchen was barren. (They gave it all away to the neighbors downstairs.) Not a single thing I had was considered edible according to their point of view. I could see where they were coming from, but then my mind started sniping at me again. *How much did all of this cost me? Oh, my God, there's nothing left. They cleaned me out. What will I snack on?*

When they made a move to trash my microwave oven, I objected. "What!" Why do I need to get rid of that?" Since I didn't have anything at all left in my kitchen to even put in a microwave oven, they said I didn't need it anymore. Of course, they were right, but I drew the line at giving away a perfectly good appliance and they backed off.

I began to realize that my attachment to food was like my attachment to negative thinking, sex, and mind-altering substances. My admission to Ryland that I wanted to fall in love one more time before I died was yet another expression of this addiction—I was still looking for something external to soothe the internal. Love was a hunger I was trying to satiate, and my lack of self-love always brought me back to food. "While overeating would be seen by some as an indulgence of self," Marianne Williamson wrote in *A Course in Weight Loss* (2010, 145), "it is in fact a profound rejection of self. It is a moment of self-betrayal and self-punishment, and anything but a commitment to one's own well-being. Why would you be able to commit to a diet if you're not consistently committed to yourself?"

In terms of my physical health, I just wanted to look good naked. In my mind, that translated into feeling good about myself. I thought that if I looked good, love would find me; ergo, feeling good naked equals happiness. That's the simplistic equation of a basic human delusion. (Buddhists talk about 108 delusions that trip us up, along with 108 desires and 108 lies we tell ourselves. Over the course of a year, that works out to a spiritual deception every day for 324 days, with 39 days for a metaphysical vacation.) Being obsessed with body image and weight is a universal, gender-neutral, equal-opportunity neurosis. Women may talk more openly about it, but men have serious body issues as well.

Since I was done with drugs, booze, and womanizing, Indian buffet restaurants had become my new bordello. Food was my surrogate high, and now I was obsessing about how even that thrill was being taken away from me . . . and to compound my anxiety, *I had voluntarily signed up for it! What was I thinking?*

3

Blowouts and Blowups, Week Two

When they informed me that a woman would stick a plastic tube up my ass and repeatedly fill me with water as part of my coaches' vision for my good health, my reactions were decidedly mixed, to put it kindly. Getting a prostate exam or a colonoscopy struck me as legitimate medical procedures designed to detect cancer. Therefore, I could tolerate that sort of discomfort if it meant keeping me healthy and alive longer, especially when performed by an anonymous male physician.

The thought of a young woman—an attractive one, at that—snaking a plastic garden hose up my backside and roto-rootering around in there filled me with trepidation. I had a vague understanding of colonics not unlike my concept of quantum physics. They said the procedure would remove harmful toxins from the walls of the intestinal tract. *Is this even a legitimate procedure? Is it anything more than just a big glorified enema? Am I going to embarrass myself?*

I imagine that a woman might experience similar feelings going to see a male gynecologist for the first time. My introduction to the colon hydrotherapist, Shayla, immediately triggered shyness and apprehension. *I don't want to be naked in front of her. I can't show this chick my ass. I'm too fat. I might have an accident on the table.* Despite my reservations,

I undressed and dutifully heaved myself atop a low platform resembling a massage table and draped a white sheet over my naked walrus carcass.

"So, Frank, I know you're nervous, but I've done thousands of sessions since 1992," said Shayla, trying to calm me. "Every single first-time client always says at the end of the session, 'That was no big deal.'"

"The nerve-racking thing isn't necessarily the mechanics of it," I replied. "It's actually showing you my ass. That's really quite disturbing, because there's no way you can get around it. You can put as much guru imagery around on the walls as you want, but at some point you've got to look at my ass and that's disturbing to me."

Shayla got down to business. "Whenever you're ready, please roll onto your left side."

"She says that like a stewardess," I joked, flopping myself into the proper position.

"Prepare for takeoff," she bantered. "And, you know, some men do think this is what it must be like to have a child. But women say it's more like menstrual cramps."

Permit me this brief digression. I later learned that the world is divided in opinion about the usefulness of what I was about to undergo. Some are big fans of colonics. Others won't put any object "where the sun doesn't shine." It turns out that colonics have an illustrious history in the Pantheon of Cleanse: Before modern medicine advocated more radical and *lucrative* procedures such as colostomy surgery and laxatives, colonics (otherwise known as the vaguely horticultural-sounding "colon irrigation") had been lightening peoples' loads for millennia. For thousands of years colonics were the sine qua non of purification. Ancient Egyptians gave themselves colonics in rivers using hollow reeds. Other Africans reaped the benefits with cow horns. The Greeks and Romans were zealous practitioners, and so were a bunch of French kings. (King Louis XIV is reported to have had over two thousand during his reign. Other French kings received court functionaries while getting the procedure, or had colonics administered to their dogs, inlaying their "clyster bags" with mother-of-pearl.) Even the explorers Lewis and Clark had one good colon cleanse on the advice of their official doctor before setting off to discover the West. Presumably, it made for happier trails.

It didn't seem like the little tube inserted into me would accommodate what would come out. While I could see everything being flushed, streaming through the tube, I was so toxic and backed up that very little came out at first other than a bunch of bubbles and some floating stringy things. "Lots of gas leaving," Shayla remarked at one point. "Do you want the thumper?"

"The what?" I exclaimed with alarm.

"The thumper," Shayla repeated, holding up a large device that resembled a serious vibrator. An abdominal massager to release stress caused by water buildup in the colon, the sound of it when turned on resembled a small propeller plane taking off.

"This is a vibrator for much older women," I tried to joke. She pointed to a switch that gave it even more power. It sounded like an outboard motor was in the room.

It all lasted less than an hour, with water repeatedly hosed in and then released. I was so incredibly self-conscious and disoriented that I just wanted it to be over quickly. It was a memorable experience, though not quite what I expected. No matter how delicately I try to explain this, it feels like an avalanche coming out of your butt. Or like El Niño and Katrina mixed into one. You get these rumbling feelings in your stomach, and you don't know what's going to happen. Next thing you know, a volcano erupts. Not normally the kind of experience I would share even with my own brother, here I was, exposing myself on film.

The next morning one of the amigos placed this message on my voicemail: "Hey, Frankie. This is Cary. I'm just calling to see if you have pooped yet today. I was hoping to be over there for the first BM. Looking forward to some colloidal plaque. Let us know if it comes out. Definitely do not flush it. I want to get over there to take some shots. Give us a call back so we can be there for that big event."

Later, Ryland followed up with me in person, asking questions like he was the Sherlock Holmes of poop. "What did the bowel movements look like?"

"Do you really want to know?" I was incredulous.

"Yeah, I want to know!" replied Ryland.

"It was some weird, web-string shit came out of me. I don't know what it was, and I don't want to know. It looked like fishing line or something. It's like my body is having a nervous breakdown."

The boys' unbridled enthusiasm about examining my first post-colonic bowel movement, to make sure it had the proper "colloidal plaque" in it, was rather unnerving and yet charming in a strange sort of way. *Such dedication, such commitment from these kids, and all of it being done in the name of improving my health. I should be beaming like a proud papa. But I'm not. I'm feeling more and more lost in this new world.*

E.T. needed to phone home. *Where is home? Could it be the eighteen inches between my head and my heart?* Every day was an exercise in surrender. Otherwise, my resistance would be about as triumphant as Custer at the Little Bighorn or Crockett at the Alamo. I was trying to cope with uncertainty. I was curious and scared at the same time.

Swept Away on a Magical Mystery Tour

Mainstream medical authorities claim there is no verifiable benefit to having your bowels flushed out. They say the benefits attributed to the procedure, such as a heightened level of energy and clarity, are a product of the imagination and just a placebo effect. My experience indicated otherwise. (By the way, I think the placebo effect is highly underrated.)

After my second colonic with Shayla, things started to get a little weird. I felt like I had been possessed by the spirit of Shirley MacLaine—an unusual compulsion came over me and I felt this surge of energy. I took a brisk walk to the nearby hardware store on Castro Street. Not understanding or caring why, I searched out an aisle of art supplies and began pulling things off the shelves. I purchased bottles and tubes of paint, of every imaginable color, along with brushes and a palette. I loaded it up and marched back to my apartment as if I were on a secret mission.

I had no idea why I was doing this. I'd never felt a compulsion in adulthood to express anything artistically through painting. I'd certainly never had any creative talent that I knew of. As soon as I got to my apartment I took everything out of the bags and just stared at this mountain of art supplies. *What am I doing? What has come over me?* Then, as if on automatic pilot, I started spontaneously painting all my kitchen cupboards in a series of swirly, multi-colored designs. No rhyme or reason to it. I was acting like Martha Stewart on acid. *Who is this guy?*

Images from kindergarten began to flash in my head. I used to love finger painting as well as using a brush. I recalled the sound of the brush against the paper. When the teacher asked me why I liked to paint, I replied that I liked the way it felt when the paint spread on the paper. She said that was a stupid reason to be painting. I should have ignored her, but instead I stopped painting. They say that sticks and stones may break your bones, but words can never hurt you. Bullshit! Words can cut deeper than a knife. My childhood was filled with incidents like that, and most left lasting scars.

What I was doing to my apartment seemed like a really good idea at the time. I must have had an unconscious desire to brighten up my surroundings. As if guided by invisible angels, I painted unusual shapes on the kitchen cabinets and on the walls, all of them swirls and colorful designs that pleased me. My brush was a conductor's wand painting a series of sensual and voluptuous curves everywhere. I had not done anything like this since kindergarten. By the day's end I had splattered paint on my arms, forehead, and hair and wore it like a badge of honor—it felt good to see it on me. I walked around the streets like that, paint spots on my clothing, paint on my shoes. I didn't care. *Who is this guy, really?*

Over the next several weeks my canvas expanded from the kitchen to my bathroom, bedroom, and living room. I was painting my heart out. I went from feeling worthless and lifeless to experiencing fleeting glimpses of contentment and happiness. I actually started to feel hope again, which replaced the dreary inner landscape I had grown accustomed to. Until recently, only the university had provided respite, especially since that semester I had been studying Gandhi and the Impressionists. Apparently in need of more nurturing, I took on painting my surroundings as a way to be myself, or rediscover a part of my authentic self. I wasn't just *doing* something. I was *awakening* to something.

My inner critical voice started to become manageable as I painted, even though it still popped up every once in a while to snipe at me. *What do you think you're doing? What's this, you think you're a painter now? You're ugly and fat! You're still an idiot!* The voice quieted as I continued painting. Rather than let it take over, I was able to be a neutral observer of my thoughts. They didn't go away entirely, but the volume toned down. I hadn't been able to do that prior to unleashing my inner Leonardo.

My landlady went ape-shit when she saw how I had painted the entire apartment. I ended up losing my $1,400 deposit even after I repainted everything to her specifications. She was angry that I hadn't asked her, and I suppose I can't blame her. She probably thought I'd gone crazy. The three amigos didn't really comment when they saw what I had created, though I could tell they felt encouraged if not amused by this turn of events.

The echo of that now familiar mantra, "this will change your life," accompanied me as I painted. Initially, it was nothing more than a slogan and New Age vapor to me. I thought my coaches were just blowing rainbows up my ass, but now I wasn't so sure. Something was certainly shifting in me, and it wasn't just my bowels.

Roto-Rootering My Toxic Thoughts

Affirmations occurred three times a day, and I hated doing them . . . *I hated them.* My coaches met with me at mealtime. I did the affirmations just before drinking the wheatgrass. Each time I felt as if I were gagging on my old life and all of my previously toxic ways. I was feeling every second of my misspent youth.

Each day, for five or ten minutes, we did some exercises out of Café Gratitude's workbook, *Abounding River*, which basically promotes the goal of being a good human. Written by Matthew and Terces, its verbiage and themes contained a hint of Landmark Forum personal development workshops. Having known that just about everyone working at Café

Gratitude had completed this group awareness program, which was an outgrowth of Werner Erhard's *est* seminars, I should not have been surprised by its influence on the restaurant's menu, workbook language, and overall approach to life.

All three of the amigos had done advanced Landmark Forum training, with a focus on developing personal and communication skills. All three of them, coincidentally or not, also came from stable, functional families. I assume that their training must have indirectly helped me because it gave them a certain vision and a support group to conduct their experiment with me. If you haven't done any personal development work on yourself, gone to AA, been in therapy, or attended similar self-development workshops or activities, Landmark Forum might be a useful place to start your road to self-discovery. But be cautious. Personally, it's not my cup of tea as I find their marketing offensive. In my opinion, after having done the Forum twice, Landmark Forum is a perpetual self-help machine. To each his own.

"Do you get that the workbook is just as important as the food?" Conor said to me at one point, with his usual youthful exuberance. "It's going to support you mentally, and your clarity and your energy." While I didn't disagree with Conor, I still felt that, to me, the affirmations, in and of themselves, were meaningless unless done in concert with other practices such as eating properly and choosing to engage in positive relationships, etc. At that point the affirmations possibly could become a catalyst for change. It then dawned on me that all of the lifestyle changes and practices they had me doing were synergy at work, leading to a transformative experience.

Eating raw food also struck me as meaningless if the rest of your life is screwed up and you are a cruel person. Adolf Hitler was a vegetarian, and that didn't seem to diminish his appetite for cruelty. Veganism does seem to at least make an honest attempt to create a holistic life experience. Once seen as a radical fringe movement, its roots go back to the ancient Greeks, Pythagoras, and the ancient healers of India. It differs from vegetarianism in its exclusion of dairy products and eggs. Today being vegan means not only eating a diet super-charged in raw, living power nutrients, it also means advocating nonviolence and exalting the beauty and preciousness of life and all sentient beings.

I used to think raw food consisted of carrot sticks, celery, and ranch dressing. Ryland explained that "Café Gratitude is a vegan, organic, mostly raw food restaurant. Raw food is vegetables, fruit, nuts, and seeds that you don't heat up above a hundred and eighteen degrees, such that the enzymatic life in that food does not die and it's still living and it has all its full nutrition." That information didn't have meaning for me at that time. So I read reams of medical science studies showing how eating raw foods can be a real bonanza for your health, particularly if you have cancer and other serious health conditions.

For Ryland and his friends, working at Café Gratitude was more than just a job or an opportunity to champion the virtues of veganism. It was a lifestyle statement. It was a platform from which they could, in Ryland's words, "deliver my life purpose and support other people in getting their greatness."

These sentiments sounded naive and idealistic to me, yet I had to extend my admiration to them. The level of commitment these guys expressed looked and felt amazing. It was still hard for me to believe they were so young and so inspired. At their age my focus in life had been consumed with drugs, sex, and rocking and rolling myself into an early grave.

Stumbling Over the Café Gratitude Steps

I was asked to work with six ways of being: Creation, Self Worth, Love and Acceptance, Gratitude, Generosity, and Abundance. It sounded like AA, therapy, and quotes from the Dalai Lama.

Matthew and the amigos further explained how I could benefit by practicing those ways of being. They urged me to take on the practice of being someone who loves my life just the way it is, right now. The boys wanted to help me become someone who could look in the mirror and say "I love and adore myself" and mean it. *That's certainly not happening yet.* They encouraged me to be someone who accepts the world as it is, which is to accept the way people are and the way that people aren't. *The 12 Steps and Buddhism have given me invaluable tools to deal with resentments.*

They asked me to be someone who is generous and grateful every single day and take that on as a conscious practice because you can't just sit around and wait for that feeling to miraculously show up. That is what the 12 Steps of AA are all about—taking action. Finally, they wanted me to practice being aware of how much of my own actions and those of others were working on my behalf, right now. I began to see how I was attached to my negative mantras, and how quick I was to defend their legitimacy.

At the end of the first week I met with Matthew to discuss abundance. Conor was also in attendance. Matthew started the session: "This quote is from Lao Tzu, and it says, 'When you realize nothing is lacking, the whole world belongs to you.' Make a list of three things you want most in your life."

That was a question I didn't need to ponder. "I want a loving relationship with my daughter. I want a PhD. And I want to be able to be of maximum service to the world, to mankind. I want to be of service."

"What would your experience be if you had all three? In other words, how would you feel about yourself? What would the experience of yourself be?"

"I think I wouldn't think about it. I think I would be in that place where I wouldn't think about how I feel. I would be okay with just being."

Matthew continued his barrage of questions, "So what would the experience be when you're not thinking?"

"Fulfilled," I replied.

"Fulfilled. Great. So practice being fulfilled now."

"Okay," I said, just to play along, but I'm really thinking, *What the hell is he talking about?*

"Close your eyes and practice being fulfilled," Matthew continued. "Throughout the day, stop and practice being fulfilled. You are the one who creates whether you are fulfilled or not. You get that?"

"Fulfilled, it just is. It is or it isn't."

"Do you get that it's a choice?" said Matthew. "There are a lot of people who have relationships with their daughters. Who have PhDs. Who make a difference in the world, and yet who aren't fulfilled. But can you get that it's just a moment-to-moment choice?"

"Yeah." *This is beginning to make some sense.*

"Can you choose being fulfilled right now?"

"Yeah." I nodded my head in agreement.

"That's it."

"It's actually easier than I thought."

"You repeat after me," Matthew instructed. "I, Frank."

"I, Frank."

And so I continued parroting Matthew, feeling like a kid who had been kept after school by his teacher to write on the blackboard a hundred times, "I will not shit all over myself in public, I will not shit all over myself in public."

"Do love me."

"My body's vigor."

"I am perfect health."

"I'm a perfect human being."

"Radiant breath."

"Raaaaaadiant beauty."

"I am divine energy."

Conor chimed in at this point, and I repeated what he said.

"I am divine." I'm having a real problem with this and having trouble taking myself seriously. "Not the guy in the movie," I tried to joke, referring to the transvestite character in a John Waters film.

"No, come on," Conor objected. "You can do this!"

"Are you talking to me?" I tried doing my best Robert De Niro impression, but neither Matthew nor Conor was buying it.

"This feels terrible," I confessed.

"You can't do the comedy thing to waver the impact," Conor scolded.

"Alright, alright." I used humor as a defense mechanism when feelings came up that I had trouble acknowledging or expressing. I thought this exercise was a sham because I felt like a fraud repeating statements I didn't believe to be true . . . at least not yet.

"I now hold in my mind this new image of myself," I repeated Conor's words, trying to finish up as fast as possible. "As a thriving, flourishing, gloriously beautiful person." You can't imagine how relieved I was every time this exercise was over.

What I didn't realize at the time, not that it would have made a difference in how I felt about it, was how much the practice of affirmations had been studied by psychologists. It wasn't just something quaint and cute to do. In scientific publications, such as the *Journal of Personal and Social Psychology*, *Psychological Science*, and *Health Psychology*, studies have shown that expressing gratitude (particularly through the use of affirmations) can greatly benefit health. It seems that counting your blessings by affirming a sense of positive self not only affects your mood, your outlook on life, and your relationships in positive ways, but it also helps relieve the symptoms of health conditions such as neuromuscular disease and chronic pain. This phenomenon is documented in experiments in which eighty-five people in a self-affirmation group were compared to a control group. Urine samples taken before and after stressful situations, such as taking an exam, showed that affirmations significantly reduced the generation of stress hormones. When you reduce stress, you improve your health.

Expressing gratitude through affirmations can yield amazing results. Nevertheless, my discomfort was so intense, I would have dismissed their significance just the same. It was like taking terrible-tasting medicine and being told how good it is for you. You aren't really ready to take it until you break down.

My "Great Detox" was well underway, and the affirmations and the colonics were a small but important part of it. In fact, everything together—the colonics, the affirmations, the diet, constantly being around positive people—was slowly opening me up, letting me see beyond my self-imposed boundaries. My awareness about the toxic patterns that characterized my life was heightening, and my body was responding to lifestyle changes along with the shift in my thought patterns.

Even though I was losing weight and gaining self-confidence, my emotional addictions and afflictions still ran deep. Those shadows were always lurking under the surface like malevolent demons masquerading as friends. The detox of my fridge, my colon, and my closet was nothing compared to the purge that needed to happen in the most complicated region of my personal geography: my mind.

4

Grief and Resolutions, Week Three

A t the center of the small, dimly lit room stood a massage table; in the background, soft New Age-y flute music whispered in the air. Part of the experiment involved deep tissue massage and aromatherapy. Bottles of essential oils lined the shelves of cabinets in the room. Massage I could handle, but this aromatherapy nonsense seemed to be going a little too far. My inner critic was alert.

I had expected a female massage therapist; instead in walked a thirty-something muscular Russian guy. "Here is the towel," he said to me in accented English. "Get undressed and on the table. I'll be right back."

Having previously seen this particular massage therapist eating at Café Gratitude accompanied by his male partner, I knew his sexual orientation. I'd never been massaged by a guy before, much less a gay guy, and I felt a wave of apprehension wash over me. *What is going on? Where is this feeling coming from?* I started telling myself there was no reason to be uncomfortable. It's no big deal. But I still felt apprehensive, and I was disturbed by my own discomfort. I'd never felt threatened or uncomfortable like this before. *This is a professional situation. I just need to relax and release this fear.* Another thought gripped me as well. *Maybe there is something in my childhood, a place I don't want to go.*

When the masseur returned, I was lying on my back under the sheet. As he began working on me I started to let go of the discomfort. After a few minutes, I relaxed and became an observer of my mind rather than a manipulator of my thoughts. When I turned over, he began massaging a spot between my shoulder blades—suddenly, Technicolor memories flooded my mind. It was like I was watching a movie of my life, similar to what people report during near-death experiences.

In this memory we were young boys fighting. I was angry, nasty, and hateful toward my younger brother, Izzy. He was trying to get away from me, and, with everything I had, I threw a punch between his shoulder blades that knocked him down and left him crying. I loved my brother, but instead of protecting him like big brothers should, I often hurt him. I turned him on to drugs when we were teens, and together we were partners in crime. I was older, I was meaner, and I had major axes to grind. I punched his back really hard, then I carried on with life and had not thought about that moment until I was lying there on that massage table over forty years later.

Consumed with sadness and remorse, I recognized that the same place I had hit my brother was where I had been experiencing debilitating spasms for years. No amount of chiropractic work or massage had been able to alleviate that familiar pain between my shoulder blades.

After the massage, the masseur wrapped me in warm blankets with only my blindfolded head exposed. I felt like a burrito lying there in stillness. An essential oil soaked into a warm cloth was gently applied to my face. I drifted into twilight sleep. More images swept over me, predominantly those of my brother. Other indistinct memories of the past contributed to a deepening sadness.

After the session, I got dressed and slumped into a chair feeling dazed. Ryland saw the distress in my face. "What's going on with you?" he asked.

"I'm feeling very sad." I replied.

"What's going on?"

"I was just thinking about a time I beat up my brother. I hit him so hard, and I wanted to hurt him. And all my life, I've had a pain in my back. The same place that I punched him. I always felt bad about it. I just didn't know how bad I felt about it. I never knew I felt bad enough to carry it all. Because I've had spasms there all my life, since that time. But I never associated it. I never associated that. I never associated that it was part of my regret for having been so cruel to my brother."

I feared the depth of anguish I held inside, but the emotional dam broke. I began sobbing shamelessly and uncontrollably, with spasms of deep, ancient sorrow and streams of un-cried tears.

"I don't think that the pain you cause other people can be separated from the pain that you incur on yourself," I said to Ryland when I regained my composure. "It's the same thing. It just never occurred to me. I would say it, but I didn't know it until just now. I didn't know that every time I took something from somebody that didn't belong to me, that I was actually robbing myself. I just didn't know. I'm sorry. I mean I'm greatly sorry. I'm really sorry I did that to him. I'm sorry I hurt a lot of people, but him in particular."

"So great, Frank," said Ryland. "This is so you showing up."

"Ughhh, God." *If this is the real me, I should throw myself under a train.*

"This is like everything I had envisioned for you. This realization. You allowing yourself to speak your truth and just rid yourself of the front. It's like so beautiful."

"I can't wait to just give him [Izzy] something that he would just never in a million years expect. And that I can barely afford. God, that sounds so fucking sappy, but on a spiritual plane, I have more and I could totally afford it. I want him to have something that he'll really love. God, this sucks, man."

I had never associated the pain in my back with my treatment of Izzy and realized, in a visceral way, that this pocket of pain lodged in my back was where I'd stored my regret at having been cruel to my brother that day. It was the subconscious dwelling of remorse. There it was, irrefutable proof that the pain you impose on others is inseparable from the pain you inflict on yourself.

I learned that what I had experienced was "somatic" release. Somatic body-oriented therapy addresses the storage of traumatic memories in our bodies. A deep tissue massage, or a session with a practitioner of somatic psychotherapy, can trigger the release of these traumas. A pioneer in this field is Peter A. Levine, PhD, who used it in his medical practice. He believed that trauma in childhood, particularly cruelty and neglect, left its marks on the body. Later in life many of these traumatized kids self-medicate with alcohol and drugs. I could relate to that. In Dr. Levine's words, they're just trying "to stabilize or suppress symptoms associated with the trauma they experienced." He also explains that "body sensation rather than intense emotion is the key to healing trauma. . . . [I]n the healing of trauma, a transformation takes place—one that can improve the quality of life" (1997, 12). In my experience to heal the wounds of emotional trauma in the body you need either somatic massage or maybe movement therapy of some kind, like dancing yourself into a wild frenzy. It's a mind and body sort of thing.

An emotional inventory of my experience on the massage table afforded me the opportunity to move on. It was like the clock on the mantle stopped at that moment, and I was allowed to go back and reset it. Just one incident on a lifelong journey, there was much more to do, and much more to discover and release.

I had cultivated a deep skepticism about aromatherapy and massage. It had all seemed silly and frivolous to me, the spiritual equivalent of snake oil. Aromatherapy, in particular, had struck me as something only wealthy women in Marin County do because they have too much time on their hands. *I was wrong. There is something to this.* It was beginning to dawn on me that I could be wrong about much more than I was willing to admit. I started doubting my arrogant certainty about things I really knew nothing about. It occurred to me that I had oceans of knowledge and only drops of wisdom.

I had heard about Rolfing and cellular memory before the massage but gave it no credence. Later, when I learned about somatics in some detail, I understood that there are issues lodged in your body that can be accessed physically through somatic or deep tissue massage. As such, the trauma, and emotional knots to be released, can be taken out by physical contact.

Nevertheless, this event alone didn't solve all of my emotional problems. It just removed a large piece of shrapnel from my back and made me aware that there was more work to be done. No matter how thorough the surgeon may be, fragments always remain. The body's natural tendency is to expel them. If you're living your life consciously, these pieces eventually make their way to the surface. It will hurt a bit, but it won't kill you.

You cannot separate the wave from the ocean.

You reap what you sow.

These maxims are at the core of every great theological principle and made up a simple but profound revelation for me: The body has a cellular memory. With this understanding, I gradually became aware of other corrosive experiences I carried around in my body. Eventually, I would come to believe this process was a component of the invisible engine driving my enduring weight loss and personal transformation.

One of my first decisions in the aftermath of that life-changing massage and aromatherapy experience was to make a vow. I would make it right with my brother, first and foremost. It was clear that I needed to go beyond my comfort zone, well beyond the act of saying, "I am sorry." I had to do something meaningful, a demonstration of love.

Setting Things Right

A few days after that gut-wrenching and unexpected massage experience I knew what I needed to do. Izzy would soon be visiting me in San Francisco from his home in New York. I already owned something that felt like it would be an appropriate gift—a Honda touring motorcycle I had purchased just a few months earlier. Izzy was a motorcycle guy and had been in a biker club when he was younger. Since he no longer had his own bike, my mission was clear. I felt that "I'm sorry" was inadequate. Love is a verb.

When Izzy and I got together at my apartment, apologizing felt much more awkward than I expected. It was hard to allow myself to be so vulnerable with him. I started off by trying to explain what I felt when the massage therapist touched the middle of my back.

"And all of a sudden it was like danger was around me," I said, dramatizing the moment. "Like all these things going 'danger, Will Robinson.' He unleashed something."

Izzy thought that was funny. But I was just getting to the serious stuff.

"Then, I started to think about all the other things. You know, like all the shitty things that I did. First of all, I gave you your first shot of dope." I continued, "You know that thing with Nancy. I always felt really bad about that."

"So did she!" Izzy shot back. He obviously hadn't forgotten the incident.

"I hooked up with a girl that you really cared about. And shit like that really corrodes the soul. It just corrodes the soul. And yet, when I got arrested, you still scrambled all over the place to come get me out of jail."

"You going to let your brother stay in jail?" Izzy shrugged like it was no big deal. Watching each other's back is what brothers are supposed to do.

"I've always felt bad about, you know, you taking care of Mom all by yourself. Without any help from me. I always wanted to apologize for anything that I ever did that hurt you. Even though it was drug induced or drug inspired or confusion. Or whatever it was, Izzy, I'm just trying to tell you . . ."

"Go ahead."

"That I apologize . . . I apologize for all the shitty things that I ever did to you. When I was supposed to be looking out for you, there I was, beating you up or giving you dope. And for all of that, I truly apologize. If you let me, I'd like to make it up to you." Izzy had just undergone eye surgery. One eye was bloodshot, and he had two black eyes. He looked like I had beaten him up just before our conversation. He stared back at me, not quite comprehending. We went downstairs and stood next to the garage. "What I want you to do is close your eye, unless your other eye works. Close both of them."

"What am I doing, Frankie? What are *you* doing?" Izzy protested.

"Alright, close your eyes. Just keep them closed." I removed the blue plastic tarp covering the polished motorcycle. "Okay, open your eyes."

Izzy stared at the motorcycle, still not sure what was happening.

"And what am I supposed to do with this?" exclaimed Izzy.

"Take it home."

"They won't take this in the baggage compartment," said Izzy, motioning toward the bike.

"Okay, you can open this then," I said, presenting him with the box my son Nick had brought over. Inside was a motorcycle jacket, leather riding gloves, and a helmet.

"Holy Jesus, what are you doing? It's not my frigging birthday."

"Open this."

"Oh, my God, this isn't just a jacket, this is a suit! This is a fucking suit, Frankie."

"You could ride through ice with this."

"Oh, Jesus." Izzy was at a loss for words. I don't know if he was more surprised or more baffled by what was going on.

"Try it on."

"Ah, look out Frisco." He got on the bike and took off riding down the steep San Francisco hills. "How am I going to get it home?" he wanted to know after his test drive.

"I'm going to ship it, I've already looked into it," I assured him.

It was an expensive way to make amends. It was also priceless. Izzy deserved it. He deserved a lot more for what I had put him through while we were growing up. This was just a karmic down payment.

You Can Go Home Again

By now I was well into my forty-two-day experiment. I'd lost an average of a pound a day. Looking down at myself I caught a glimpse of my foreskin—a momentous occasion. For years I had only seen it in a mirror.

I felt energetic. I'd cleaned out lots of chaos in my head, and people told me I looked radiant. (Not feeling like you want to die really helps a guy look better.) Though I continued to carve out new neural pathways, of all the things I'd experienced—the raw food regimen, the affirmations and the bodywork, the come-to-Jesus moments on the weight scale, and the unlikely camaraderie I enjoyed with my three unrelenting young agents of change—nothing compared to confronting the weight I'd carried literally and symbolically on my back.

Marianne Williamson wrote that integral to weight loss is the importance of reestablishing "the divine connection that was severed by any harshness in your childhood" (2010, 147). That includes harshness done unto you or harshness that you've done to others, which is to say that forgiveness of self and others is an integral component to wellness. It's a long road from psychic rupture to psychic rapture.

My wellness assessments, in the physical realm, occurred periodically over the six weeks with visits to naturopathic physicians and nutritionists, in addition to visits to my usual hepatitis C doctors. These sessions were markers charting how far I had come and how much farther I had to go. One of those sessions was with Anusha Amen-Ra, nutritionist and director of Sacred Space Retreat Center, and what he explained to me was both enlightening and something no medical authority had ever told me.

"We're going to take a quick look here at your blood," said Amen-Ra. "This is what we call a live blood analysis in which we're using a dark field microscope. So one of the first things that I'm seeing here is you've got some bacteria forms that are in your protoplasm. You probably have a serious issue with yeast overgrowth. Anybody that has cancer or any other kind of major disease, long before you get that, twenty, thirty, forty years before, you start having issues with yeast overgrowth. Frank, you have all of the issues of illness that are appropriate for someone who eats the way you have."

Amen-Ra went on to explain that my reliance on eating mostly cooked food along with processed and fast food over the years meant that I had been digesting pabulum devoid of essential enzymes and lacking proper nutrition. Essentially, the high heat from cooking tends to kill off most of the nutrients we humans require to keep our immune system healthy.

My visits for medical evaluations by Dr. Joel, a holistic practitioner, mostly involved answering his questions and acknowledging the obvious—I am overweight, my hepatitis C contributes to my fatigue, and I take too many prescription medications.

I explained that in 2001 prior to my diagnosis, I went through a battery of tests to try to establish why I was so tired all the time. My doctors, who hadn't found the hepatitis C at first, were treating me for narcolepsy, and I was given a prescription for Provigil, a strong drug usually given to patients with narcolepsy, to help me stay awake.

After the hepatitis C diagnosis, my doctor put me on a cocktail of drugs that I was told were a form of chemotherapy, similar to what women with breast cancer are prescribed. I took capsules of one of the drugs every day and an injection of the other every week. To counter the side effects of these drugs, I was prescribed a slew of other medications. Among the side effects were depression, fatigue, achy joints, irritability, and poor sleep. The problem with taking meds is that the doctor's answer to every subsequent issue is another pill.

Every morning I took a fistful of pills and didn't really know what they were doing to me. I had no idea how they were interacting with each other inside me or if they were creating more health problems. Doctors were telling me to take them, so I took them.

I felt trapped in a hopeless cycle: If I felt sad, I wasn't sure if it was causal or because the medications needed redialing. It was an awful and difficult place. The sad fact is that many people face similar health dilemmas. I took solace from knowing I wasn't alone in the insane web of mainstream medicine.

The harsh reality was that my health situation existed because of the way I played the cards I was dealt—the decisions I made to use drugs, legal and illegal, ripping and running and carrying on like there was no tomorrow. I was one of the fortunate. My health could have been much worse. I could have been infected with HIV, or contracted any number of other serious conditions due to my lifestyle and behaviors. Miraculously, I had survived the sixties and the eighties.

But I wasn't feeling the luck. I wasn't feeling the gratitude either. I kept thinking, hoping, that a shift was coming. Somewhere in me I believed that things would change for the better. I just couldn't see how that was going to happen. Beneath the surface this experiment was beginning to change all of that.

"When were you diagnosed with hepatitis C?" asked Dr. Joel.

"About four or five years ago."

"You're taking the Effexor too? Provigil? And Ribavirin?"

"Right."

"Are you taking any nutritional supplements?"

"No, and I'll tell you why," I replied. "I don't take them because I don't know who to believe. If I speak to four doctors about vitamins and supplements, I have one that tells me they're useless. One will tell me you'll die if you don't take them. The other one says just take this one. And the last one says it's all bullshit. These are all guys with the same diploma. So I don't know what to do."

Dr. Joel didn't argue with me. He already had some supplement suggestions in mind. "How is your libido? Your sex drive?"

"I have none at the moment," I had to confess. "I haven't had sex since I don't know when. I don't even remember the last time I saw my dick. Which is really a crime for a warm-blooded Sicilian guy like myself, who is full of poetry and romance."

Not a laugh, not even a smile creased Dr. Joel's lips. This guy was all business, and my attempts at humor bounced off him like pebbles against a tank. It was just as well. I was beginning to question everything I thought I was sure about, including what the mainstream doctors had told me. I felt like I landed on a new planet, strolling through uncharted territory deep within my unexamined self.

After my third visit to Dr. Joel, my mainstream doctors ran a blood test and discovered that my hepatitis C was virtually untraceable—a really momentous occasion for me after all of my battles with that ailment. Did the raw foods diet and wheatgrass contribute to my success in vanquishing hepatitis C? Maybe. I don't know. I had been on hepatitis C-treatment protocol for six months prior to filming, so it was hard to know what did what. I do know the side effects from all of the medications diminished a great deal while I was on the raw foods diet. I felt more energetic, more hopeful and optimistic. I went from waking up thinking, *oh, shit, another fucking day* to thinking *oh, boy, I wonder what will happen today*.

The mainstream doctors asked me to continue taking the medications for another three months to keep the hepatitis C from returning. I agreed to do that, and this sheep-like acquiescence on my part would prove to be a big mistake. (More on that turn of events later.)

Call Me Raw Friendly

Café Gratitude's menu was mostly raw but not strictly raw; it was, however, all vegan. During my six weeks of eating there every day I learned about the health benefits of raw foods and wheatgrass juice. I also learned how it felt to be satisfied after a meal instead of feeling stuffed and bloated.

If you have an illness or disease—which happens to most of us at some point in our lives—you might be well served to adopt a raw foods diet accompanied by wheatgrass juice. "Let food be thy medicine and medicine be thy food!" said Hippocrates. The right foods can be powerful preventive medicine even if you just want to maintain your health by keeping your immune system strong. Am I beginning to sound like an advocate?

What I found out about cooked foods surprised me. Not only does cooking destroy many of the vital nutrients in plant foods—vitamins, minerals, and phytochemicals—meats cooked at high temperatures also contain carcinogens that can weaken your immune system. The following articles regarding harmful effects of cooked foods from the hundreds I found in the medical literature are not information enough to bore you, but enough to wake you up, as it did me.

- After comparing the effects of common cooking practices— e.g., boiling, steaming, microwaving—on raw broccoli and Brussels sprouts, researchers found a large decrease in the phytochemical content of all the vegetables from all of the cooking methods; ascorbic acid (vitamin C) showed the greatest loss (Pellegrini et al. 2010).
- Scientists tested the effects of a strict uncooked vegan diet on patients with severe cases of rheumatoid arthritis and found numerous key health indicators, such as LDL cholesterol that was "significantly decreased by the vegan diet" and a relief of arthritic symptoms (Agren et al. 2001).
- A group of 239 bladder cancer patients were monitored over eight years to assess their raw broccoli consumption and cancer mortality. A "strong and significant" association was

found: Those who ate more raw broccoli, not the cooked variety, survived the longest (Tang et al. 2010).

- South American scientists discovered that "boiled meat and cooked vegetables" consumption was "directly associated with risk of oral and pharyngeal cancer." Raw vegetable consumption was found to reduce the risk of these cancers (De Stefani et al. 2005).

- German scientists matched a group of 310 women with breast cancer with an equal group of women without breast cancer and measured their intake of raw vegetables. Those who ate the most raw vegetables significantly lowered their risk for breast cancer (Adzersen et al. 2003).

- After studying thousands of people, "significant associations with colorectal cancer risk were observed for red meat, pork, and processed meat" consumption, while "significant protections" were found against colon cancer for those who ate a diet rich in raw vegetables, especially garlic (Levi et al. 1999).

After six weeks with the three amigos and exposure to Café Gratitude, I came around to being a vegan- and raw food-friendly guy. Most people don't have the discipline or commitment, and it's unrealistic to think anyone would transform into a raw foods vegan because of a few (well, really a lot more than a few) studies. What you can do to dramatically improve your health, is gradually integrate raw foods into your diet, which is what I have done.

Is Anyone Home?

On a whim, or a THC-inspired attack of genius, the boys spontaneously showed up at 2:00 a.m. at my apartment. I heard something at the front door, leaped out of bed, and grabbed a bat.

"Oh, Frank, you scared the shit out of me, man!" Cary exclaimed.

"I scared *you*?" I replied.

I thought he was wacked since I was the one who should have freaked out when my front door mysteriously opened in the middle of the night, accompanied by sneaky footsteps.

Ryland spoke up, "We decided we'd come and check in on you."

"I'm glad you did. I've been thinking about you guys. I don't know if you can tell that I feel a lot better."

"Yeah, I could tell right away," replied Cary.

"My shoulder blades are killing me. If I take more medicine, I'm afraid I'm not going to get up in the morning. By virtue of the affection I have for you guys, it's important to me to do my best. That's the only way I'll be able to forgive myself if I fuck up. But sometimes that's very hard. I'm not really sure how to do that."

"What are you afraid of?" asked Ryland.

"I'm afraid of letting you down. More than that, I'm afraid I'll just cut out. In any kind of affectionate relationship, whether it's a romantic relationship or a friendship, once you realize that you really dig the person, then you run the risk of getting hurt. This lady that I met in the restaurant tonight said something to me really very powerful, so powerful that it stopped me dead in my tracks. I almost got misty. She said, 'Love like you've never been hurt.'"

What I think she was saying was that I had to first learn how to love myself before I could learn how to unconditionally love another human being. I knew she was right. My work was certainly cut out for me.

What I heard was that I needed to practice radical forgiveness. I needed to forgive everyone for everything, and that was going to be tough. Holding on to resentments gives me a temporary sense of superiority and the surge of power that comes from righteous indignation. It's like a few shots of vodka—moments of pleasure and relief followed by weeks of remorse. Anger is stronger than fear. Anger always trumps sorrow.

5

Forgiveness and Redemption, Week Four

In order for me to make room for this new person I was cultivating, I had to make room in the space of my life. This meant letting go of stuff, at least that was what Conor proposed to me. He was congenitally full of bright ideas. "It's a kind of spiritual feng shui," Conor described my assignment.

"So what does that really mean?" I asked.

Conor and the others explained what they had in mind, and my resistance came up, big time. They wanted me to clean out my closet and give away most of my shoes and clothing, everything that I no longer wore or used. My mind churned out a series of calculations: *These clothes were expensive. I bought most of these in Washington, DC. Those are Italian shoes. How many hours did I work to buy them? What if I get rid of these clothes, and this whole experiment doesn't work?* My doubts were surging up like a tsunami. Manufacturing concerns that I might need these clothes again was just my way of clinging to a bunch of useless stuff and the old memories attached to that stuff.

Cary, Conor, and Ryland watched over me as I went through my closet, cleaning it out item by item. I remembered each item, where I bought it, what I paid, the last time I wore it, all of the telltale signs of attachment. I folded the pants, shirts, and suits and neatly placed everything from my closet into three large trash bags. The amigos helped me carry the bags down to my car and smiled as we set the bags into the trunk of my ten-year-old silver Infiniti. Their giddiness was contagious, and I started to get into the spirit of my sacrifice. We drove through San Francisco, the Stones blasting through the open windows.

I suggested we go find some homeless people, who needed clothing the most. Normally there were a lot of those pour souls hanging out south of Market Street. We embarked on an hour-long hunt for homeless people, and I swear to God we couldn't find any. The streets were eerily empty. We finally found a single group of seven or so, two of them women, milling about on a street corner. "How are you guys doing? Do you need some clothes?" I said from the car.

Maybe because the three amigos and I were in such high spirits, these folks gazed at us with apprehension. In retrospect, if I saw us, I would be suspicious, too. They finally approached the car. We bantered back and forth until they got more relaxed. The whole scene soon turned pleasant. I took all my stuff out of the trunk and displayed it. There were a dozen pairs of Italian shoes on the hood, and we let the people choose what they wanted. In that moment, it occurred to me that I had been spared their particular hardship purely by grace. That could have easily been me hanging out on that corner. In a real sense I was not just there to give away clothes, but to make a connection and look them in the eye and recognize how nothing separated me from them.

Upon leaving I noticed my initial resistance had shifted to a sense of joy. The more expensive something was the greater the pleasure in giving it away. It seemed strange to me that releasing a Neiman Marcus purchase could give me such peace. Giving it all away inspired gratitude for where I had landed in life, despite all of the challenges that still confronted me. My troubles didn't begin to compare with the mornings and nights of these people. It's really hard to be pissed off at anything or feel victimized if you feel gratitude.

The guys acknowledged me for what I had done. They saw this as a step toward positive change. "You know, the more that you allow yourself to give away, it's opening up the space for more to rush in," Ryland said to me. "You're making space in your life for all new things."

They hadn't expected me to be so compliant in giving away more than two-thirds of my clothing and shoes, and I expected to feel giver's remorse, but it never came. Those things I had given away rapidly faded from my memory, an indication of how unimportant they were. Though counterintuitive, such an activity can open you up and give you a different perspective on your entire life. It's like standing on a desk looking over the room instead of just sitting in your chair day after day.

Retrieving Memories of Joy

When I allow myself to be vulnerable, my spirit is naked and my ego screams to be covered. It's frightening for me to stand in that place within myself, yet that is where joy and authenticity breathe life into my soul. "The more real you get, the more unreal the world gets" (John Lennon).

I grew up in Brooklyn. My neighborhood consisted of blue-collar southern Italians. We had access to a small Salvation Army recreation center a block away from Knickerbocker Park. One hot summer, the center offered to take some of us to camp for two weeks. This was a big deal because it was free and hardly anyone ever left the neighborhood for too long a period of time—that is, except for the "wise guys" who went to jail or the afterlife. My mom gathered up what little money she could and took me shopping to John's Bargain Store on Knickerbocker Avenue for new underwear, T-shirts, socks, a sweater, bathing suit, sneakers, and toiletries. I felt like a rich kid with all of this new stuff.

Upon arrival at summer camp I was surprised to find some of the kids were in deeper poverty than my family. I made friends with one kid, from an exotic-sounding place called Yonkers, who described his home life as if it were a dark cavern in a dank outback. He definitely seemed to be worse off than me, and knowing his circumstances summoned something in me that I couldn't identify.

The two weeks flew by, and in spite of the slew of exciting and novel activities, my most intense memory occurred when it was time to pack up and leave. I noticed that my new friend from Yonkers only had a few rags that he was stuffing into a brown paper bag. Something about his quiet poverty moved me and hurt at the same time. Without thinking, I started handing him all of my clothing. We were about the same size, and he seemed very grateful to have it all. My gesture relieved some of my anxiety about his circumstances and made me feel better.

When the bus dropped me back in Brooklyn, I began to panic. I remembered my mother's sacrifice in scrounging up enough money so her kid could attend camp with some new clothes to wear. *She's gonna kill me*, the thought began pounding in my head. I imagined the wrath that awaited me when I walked through our apartment door. I crept up the dark stairway to the second floor; the pungent smell of vinegar wafted up from the cellar where Mr. Piccolo made his wine. My mother embraced me tightly after I walked in the door and held on as if I had just been released from the clutches of a kidnapper. Her loving enthusiasm only worsened my fear as she kissed my face over and over again then took my little suitcase over to the kitchen table and opened it up.

Oh, boy, here it comes, I thought.

She looked inside and paused. I squirmed uncomfortably. "Frankie, where is everything?"

"I'm so sorry, Mom," I blurted, on the verge of tears. "This guy in the bunk next to me; he was so poor. He was from Yonkers. He didn't have any stuff, so I gave him mine."

Mom got quiet. She sat down and began to cry. My heart sank. The last thing I wanted to do was hurt Mom or make her ashamed of me. I walked over to her, apologizing for my actions every step of the way. She reached up and embraced me.

"No, no, son," she told me. "I'm so glad you're like that. You have a heart. Don't worry about those things. What you did was right."

The relief I felt was mixed with the feeling I mentioned earlier, the one I didn't understand. It was compassion. My mother had it in abundance; she had always been extraordinarily generous, both with her emotions and material possessions. Her poverty never eroded her giving spirit—if anything, being poor had only strengthened her resolve to share what little she had and express gratitude for what little she had left. My mother taught me how to give with joy in my heart. In my addiction, I forgot what it felt like to give with an open heart, without an agenda of receiving anything in return.

In 1988, I got a job as a carpenter in a psychiatric hospital where there was no shortage of sad stories—the children's unit was the most heartbreaking with kids ranging in age from six to fourteen years. On Sundays the parents came to visit. One look at them and it was clear why the kids ended up in a nut house. Sometimes life is painfully unfair. One kid in particular, a boy about eight years old, attracted my attention. He sometimes had difficulty speaking, especially when he was upset. One day while making my rounds, I noticed him crying in frustration. After several hours the staff had given up trying to console him. They just left him standing in the same spot to shed his anguished tears.

My heart swelled with sorrow and compassion as I wondered what I could do for him. When I noticed he was standing near a water fountain, I intuitively walked over and lifted him up so he could reach it and take a drink. After taking his fill, his demeanor immediately changed, and, with a smile, he ran off down the hallway to play. Unable to verbally convey his need, he had been crying because he couldn't reach the water fountain; the boy just needed a little lift. I raced to my workshop and built the boy small, portable steps. I carved his name on the top step so he could see that he mattered to someone.

This story isn't to convey what a nice guy I am. When I saw that little boy unable to communicate his needs, I saw myself in him. Whenever something seemed out of reach to me, I always felt ashamed at my perceived inadequacy, and I would rarely ask for help. At that moment I felt divinely guided. As I ran the wood through the bench saw and assembled the pieces for the steps, I felt myself brimming with a joyful, deeper knowing. I was doing the right thing. I was fulfilled, grateful, and blessed. I had made a difference in someone's life.

Sometimes all we need is a little lift from someone who understands: The three amigos at Café Gratitude, Cary, Conor, and Ryland, felt compassion for me and gave me a lift, a really big lift that changed my life.

Gratitude Is Good for You (and Me)

You've heard the expressions "count your blessings," "blessings in disguise," and "every dark cloud has a silver lining." These notions of gratitude used to be nothing more than tired clichés to me. I've since come across a lot of impressive research on the benefits of expressing gratitude.

Gratitude is the feeling that you've received a benefit or gift provided by someone else—by another person, by God, by whatever source. "we recognize that the sources of this goodness are outside of ourselves. . . . We acknowledge that other people—or even higher powers, if you're of a spiritual mindset—gave us many gifts, big and small, to help us achieve the goodness in our lives," says Robert A. Emmons, PhD, a professor of psychology at the University of California, Davis (*Greater Good: The Science of a Meaningful Life* 2014). Among pioneering psychologists, Dr. Emmons has conducted studies on how being grateful affects us emotionally and physically. In one of his studies, Dr. Emmons asked a group of volunteers to write down what they were grateful for, while another group wrote about what was going wrong in their lives. After a few weeks, he found that the "gratitude" group had more energy and zest for life, and slept better, than those in the "complaining" group. These findings mirrored my experience during the six-week experiment—it doesn't take any creativity or courage to be pessimistic.

An attitude of gratitude—particularly in the midst of suffering—will have a positive effect on the health of body and mind. Dr. Emmons says, "Being grateful builds social relationships, for example, and studies show that people with more social support are healthier than those without it" (Emmons and Stern 2013). The three amigos' social support helped to open me up in a heartfelt way. I caught a glimpse into a new way of being.

Maybe you don't feel grateful very often. I certainly didn't. But can you consciously *develop* an attitude of gratitude? Dr. Emmons insists gratitude can be cultivated and is not a trait but a conscious choice. Affirmations, however painful or false they may feel in the moment, are one way to cultivate the benefits of gratitude in your life and are a technique for carving a new neural pathway in your brain, which certainly had an impact on me despite my resistance.

Oy! Another Irrigation

"Come right into the colonic room," said Shayla cheerfully.

"Oh, joy of joys."

Before beginning the procedure, Shayla asked me to describe the aftermath of my previous two colonics experiences: "The first one was scary because it was so new, and my abdomen was a bit sore."

"It happens to some people, but your life will change."

It will change my life. I still regarded such statements with a mild degree of skepticism if not cynicism. *These sorts of sayings are nebulous and open-ended. I take a dump and it's going to change my life? When you're feeling lousy you just want to feel better. There was just stuff stuck in my intestines.* And yet, my entire apartment had become a painter's canvas after my last colonic.

"Yeah, right," I replied. "You know what I was thinking when you told me that? I was thinking, 'Okay, I've tried so hard to change my life. This lady's going to stick a tube up my ass with some water and my life is going to change. Yeah, right.' Like everything else about the six weeks, I surrendered to it. I could hardly walk properly when I got out of here. Not from the tube, but rather from the intestinal spasms. Keep in mind I had months, maybe years, of waste lodged deep. My bowel movements were bi-weekly at best. Getting regular was like the shifting of tectonic plates. The next one was a little different. By the third one I am feeling like Shirley MacLaine lives in my house. After the last colonic I started cleaning like you would not believe. I started taking care of everything, including polishing the rims on my car! Shortly after that, I was in a hardware store and bought art supplies and started painting murals. Who is this guy? Really! Who is this guy?"

"These were things that were yearning to be expressed all along." Shayla replied matter-of-factly, as if she had heard my story from a thousand different clients.

"All because I needed to take a dump?" I said.

"No, it's more than that," she said, just above a whisper.

"Three weeks ago, I could barely walk up here because I was feeling so shitty. Now I'm feeling energetic. I'm not thinner, but I'm feeling thinner.

It's more important to feel good, than to look good. With this regimen, the food, the colonics, all of it, I'm not saying it is the answer for everyone. But it's definitely worth a try."

Not long after this last colonic I went to see Dr. Joel again. Ryland and Conor were tagging along with the camera as they had during the colonics treatments.

"I caught a glimpse of my foreskin one morning!" I told the doc. "I kind of took my stomach in, but I saw a glimpse! I can't tell you how happy I was."

"You look good," interjected Ryland.

"I think it's just not feeling like I want to die. That really helps a guy look better, you know?"

"What can you say is different about your experience of life from the last time we walked in this doctor's office?" asked Ryland.

"Simply put, seventy percent of the chaos in my head and in my life is gone. You guys are forcing me to push the envelope all the time. Goddamn it, it's exhausting. I sleep good, but I'm worried about the envelope falling off the side of the cabinet. You know what I mean? I keep pushing that bad boy."

Dr. Joel then got his turn at interrogation. "So, how are you doing since the last time I saw you? You've been doing the dieting?"

"I've been sticking to it, period. I've done three colonics. And my closets are so clean now. I'm telling you. I don't know who that guy was. It was like this dormant Virgo burst on the scene!"

"So you're feeling better in general?"

"In general, I'm feeling much better. I'm feeling much more energetic. I just feel hopeful; I feel alive. As opposed to before I just was really depressed and feeling hopeless. When I first came here, I felt fat. My stomach is the same size, but I don't feel fat."

"No shortness of breath?"

"Only when I run up the stairs."

"Gas or bloating?"

"No bloating. But gas in the sense that when you eat this stuff, man, you can raise a goddamn balloon. Not that it's unpleasant or negative. It's unpleasant for other people, but it doesn't bother me at all."

"How are your bowel movements? Are they regular?"

"My bowel movements are spectacular! They're not just good. I mean, they're really an event. Actually, they're such an event I don't even use toilet paper anymore. I just go straight to the shower."

"Okay. Are you sleeping well?"

"I'm sleeping very well."

"How's your energy level?"

"It's better, man. Are you kidding? It's like much better."

"Okay, wonderful. Your lab work was done, right?"

"The lab work that I do know about is the blood work with the hep C, and they said that there is no visible trace of it whatsoever. They just want to continue the therapy. They just want to make sure they get everything. But for all intents and purposes, I'm cured of hep C, which is really cool."

"So let's compare the results of your tests, okay?"

"It's like Mr. Rogers: 'Let's go over to the train.'"

As usual, Dr. Joel didn't crack a smile. Maybe he didn't get the joke.

I stepped on the scale, and a number materialized—264.

"Wow. What was it before? 287. This scale is fucked up. Man, wait a second."

"No, it's not lying," the doc objected.

"No kidding. No wonder I saw my foreskin. Almost a pound a day lost. Wow."

When I try to explain the six-week experiment, I find it impossible to say that one thing was responsible for the changes in me. The raw foods diet certainly had an impact on my weight. The three amigos on my case like white on rice and me forcing myself to do things that I really didn't want to do all helped me back to the person that I was supposed to be in the first place. Like peeling the layers off an onion, each teary-eyed discovery about my true nature was accompanied with the need to summon renewed commitment to finding out even more.

6

Acceptance and Healing, Week Five

Throughout my life I've harbored a deep resentment for the Catholic Church. I poured Miracle-Gro on that resentment and nurtured it to the point where it became a part of my identity. Whenever I thought of the Church, I thought of all the horrors of the Inquisition as well as my own experiences. As a child I was hit and terrorized by nuns, street pukes, cops, parents, and other authority figures claiming to be devoted Catholics and followers of Jesus. As a result, I learned to navigate through life predicated on fear instilled in me as a child. I brought these fears with me everywhere: fear that I wasn't good enough, smart enough, tall enough, handsome enough . . . fill in the blanks.

The nuns at my Catholic school were purveyors of the medieval. The place was St. Leonard School in Brooklyn, but it should have been called Our Lady of Perpetual Pain and Sorrow. The nuns' brand of punishment would have given Stalin a hard-on. These people got into a kid's head and injected a virulent level of incomprehensible fear. Their approach was holistic, their attack complete: mind, body, soul. According to them, God saw and recorded your thoughts—all your thoughts, and in Catholicism the thought is tantamount to the deed. Your body is always perched and ready for sin. If you touch yourself, Jesus and the Blessed Mother see it, and the deed would be remembered on Judgment Day—by the time I was nine years old, I knew I was condemned. My best hope was to cop a plea and get into Purgatory, but then Vatican II eliminated Purgatory and so I was doomed. Vatican II also eliminated Saint Christopher, although the wise guys kept him on their Cadillac dashboards anyway.

The fourth step in AA deals with resentments, and the Catholic Church led the hit parade. When I finally got sober, my sponsor listened patiently while I explained how cruel the nuns and priests had been and what they did to me as a child. Following my sorrowful and venomous presentation, my sponsor calmly asked what my part had been in it all. I was surprised and annoyed at the question. *How could I have played a part in my own abuse?*

As far as I was concerned, I had no part in it. I was just a victim, nothing else. I was subjected to physical abuse and emotional terrorism by agents of the Catholic Church and, by extension, God himself. The nuns would unleash cruelty with bestial ferocity: I was already worried about going to Hell before I had experienced my first French kiss. At the age of eleven, I went to confession at least once a week in case I met with a fatal car accident. I don't remember how many times I went home soiled because the nuns refused to let me go to the bathroom. The list goes on.

I had become a prisoner of these events; my experience as a child became my identity as an adult. If you had met me back then, within a few minutes I would have introduced you to this resentment and enrolled you in my army of people against the Catholic Church. My past served as a license for all my bad behavior. As I recalled these events for my sponsor, I could feel my anger rising.

I told my sponsor that I was a helpless little kid and that I had not played a part in anything. He looked at me calmly and said, "Your part is that you held on to this anger and resentment for so long. Your part in it is that you refused to let it all go." We sat together quietly for a few moments while my brain short-circuited and re-circuited. At that moment, I was compelled to look at my life through a new lens. I recognized my attachment to being a victim. Irrespective of this insight, it would take another decade before I could forgive.

Fast-forward ten years, I was going out with this woman who had an interest in Catholicism and asked me to take her to mass. She had a light-weight Protestant background, so I understood her fascination with the Catholic Church: Protestant churches tend to be rather Spartan, devoid of ritual and imagery. We visited St. Monica's, a church with enough pictures and statues of graven images to give any good Protestant a seizure. I explained the symbols and rituals to her. By the middle of mass she was completely mesmerized. She decided to become Catholic.

Knowing of my resentments toward the Church, she took it upon herself to set up an appointment for me with the Monsignor. For those of you outside the faith, a Monsignor is like middle management. "See this guy," she said. "He wants to talk to you about reconciliation."

I wanted to keep the peace, so I reluctantly agreed to go. In my mind I was sharpening my knife. I conjured up the wolf looking at the chicken. I had a long list of indictments, dating back to the 1950s. My intention was to crucify this guy—I set out to get my revenge.

The Monsignor had a well-appointed Catholic office, typical of a well-to-do diocese: huge oak crucifix, thick burgundy velvet curtains, large oak furniture upholstered with more red velvet. You couldn't steal anything from this guy's office because everything was too heavy to lift. He sat in one corner of the room, and I sat in the other. "I understand you have some issues with the Catholic Church."

I said, "Issues? Magazines have issues. I have volumes of resentments." I took a deep breath and prepared to unleash my venom. I was feeling self-righteous and indignant. Before I finished my first sentence, however, he asked me, "When was the last time you went to confession?" I was struck dumb.

I thought, *the nerve of this guy. He's got balls like grapefruits. How dare he ask me this question when I am here to indict him?* The Catholics had me conditioned as a little boy, I reflexively replied, "I don't remember the last time I went to confession."

"How about now?" he shot back. Without missing a beat, he raised his hand and with his thumb and first two fingers made the sign of the cross.

Without thinking I started saying, "Bless me, Father, for I have sinned." Suddenly on automatic pilot, I was responding like I was a kid again but as

55

an observer rather than a participant—as if I were having an out-of-body experience.

"What are your sins, my son?"

I'm thinking, *what is going on here?* But somehow I surrendered to the moment and said to him, "You know, Father, I'm not going to get into all of the tedious details of the things that I did. I did a lot that I'm not proud of. I'm sure I broke most of the Ten Commandments several times. But the one thing I feel a great deal of remorse about is that I hurt people. Sometimes I did it carelessly, sometimes inadvertently, and sometimes deliberately, but always for selfish reasons. Either way in the end the result was the same. For that I am truly sorry and feel the greatest regret."

I sank deeper into the plush velvet chair, feeling small and defeated; there was a long pause. He looked at me with profound kindness, making the sign of the cross again with his thumb and first two fingers pointing upward, and said, "My son, from the bottom of my heart and on behalf of the Catholic Church, I apologize for all of the wrongs that were done to you. I am truly sorry. In the name of the Father, the Son, and the Holy Ghost, you are forgiven and absolved of all your sins. And now, my son, I leave you to the daunting task of forgiving yourself."

I crossed myself and wept. I didn't know it at the time, but the Monsignor had just mapped out my difficult journey for many years to come. Self-forgiveness would be my Mount Everest.

I walked out of that office and into the street feeling an indescribable emptiness. I had just made peace with a part of my past. My resentments about the Catholic Church had dissolved, leaving me with the residue of my wreckage that they had obscured. A part of my identity was gone because I had so identified with my resentments.

I learned that in order to forgive myself I had to begin forgiving others, and that meant forgiving the entity of the Catholic Church as well as the nuns and priests. Shortly after my confession I traveled back to Brooklyn to visit my mother. I borrowed a car and drove to my old neighborhood.

I wanted to see St. Leonard's Church, the convent and school, that had been the source of so much of my anguish—places where children suffered. In my head, I had a deeply spiritual and slightly melodramatic letting-go ritual rattling around. When I got to the site, everything was unfamiliar. For a moment I wasn't sure where I was. The church was gone. St. Leonard's Church, a huge gothic structure, the rectory, and convent were all gone. Everything had been leveled. In their place stood an apartment complex. Except for the school building, a dreary Eastern Bloc, Stalinesque, gray concrete blight (though much smaller than I remembered), all architectural evidence of my childhood nightmare experiences was gone.

I wondered if everything in my life had been a dream wrapped in an illusion. I suddenly realized that I was the only one giving life to this memory. Every major player in my little saga had been dead a long time, but I had kept them on life support.

A part of me likes feeling resentful because it affords me the illusion of empowerment and superiority, and that feels safe. Underneath that is hurt which exposes vulnerability. Men of my generation, instead of being taught to reveal this vulnerability, were taught the opposite. The macho notion of what it means to be a man was about hardening your heart, and there are still times when I slip into that darkness. Sometimes it's not easy to get back to the light. Crack the door of willingness an inch and help will come your way in the light.

If I choose to embrace and fuel my resentments, I am spared the responsibility of releasing and embodying my better self. The payoff is the relief at not having to take responsibility for any kind of success or failure. In other words, if I choose to feel bad about myself and say that I am not smart enough, then I don't have to take the risk in writing that book or taking that class or learning how to play the instrument. Living in fear is like pouring astringent on your spirit; life shrinks when you coddle neurosis.

For most of my life I never thought that I could write a book. In fact, I still sometimes feel that I will be struck by lightning if I say I'm a writer. But if I say that I am a writer, then I have to write something. I have to do what I say in order to feel like an authentic human being. If I hide behind the mask of insecurity, then I don't have to do anything. That doesn't mean the insecurity is gone; it just means that I'm not hiding behind it as much.

My heart and mind were ultimately resuscitated by forgiveness. That doesn't mean I made "them" right or what "they" did okay. It means that by practicing forgiveness I made room in my heart for love.

P.S. Genuinely forgiving someone doesn't mean you have to take them to lunch.

Forgiveness Is Good for Your Health

Forgiveness is powerful medicine. It liberates the mind and opens the heart. An internet search under the terms "forgiveness and health" turns up several hundred medical science studies documenting how the act of forgiving someone, particularly yourself, heals illness and bestows the gifts of health.

Forgiving someone is for *your* sake, for *your* emotional healing. The genuine act of forgiveness can heal and resurrect the most fractured relationships. Holding resentments and coddling grudges can create unhealthy consequences. Forgiveness is taking responsibility for how *you* feel. Forgiveness is a proven path toward peace of mind.

Dr. Fred Luskin cofounded and directs the Stanford University Forgiveness Project. He also authored the book *Forgive for Good: A Proven Prescription for Health and Happiness* in which he explains how everyone can learn how to forgive. "Forgiveness can be taught and learned, just like learning to throw a baseball" (2014).

When I couldn't forgive or didn't want to forgive, I fostered the illusion of superiority, power, and righteousness. I was more interested in being right than in being happy. Resenting someone or something is like drinking the poison and hoping the other person dies. If you're interested in a long and healthy life, eat intelligently, exercise, and practice kindness and forgiveness. It's been documented that people who blame others for their troubles have a higher incidence of heart disease and cancer. Scientific studies have shown that people who are forgiving have fewer health problems overall, including fewer physical symptoms from stress such as high blood pressure and insomnia. "Every time you revisit a sense of grievance, you cause stress to the body," says Dr. Luskin (2014).

The following are studies showing the power of forgiveness.

Health benefits start with the heart. Forgiveness provides numerous health advantages, including "long-term buffering against cardiovascular reactivity" such as high blood pressure, as this study concluded. A group of 202 volunteer participants thought about a previous incident from either an angry or forgiving perspective and had their systolic and diastolic blood pressure and heart rate measured. During the mental recreation of the offense, practicing the use of forgiving thoughts offered sustained protection against the kind of reactivity that had physical effects detrimental to health (Larsen et al. 2012).

Forgiveness releases the pain of anger in the lower back. I could relate to this research given what happened to me on the massage table. With sixty-one patients complaining of chronic low back pain, a team of seven scientists studied levels of pain, anger, and psychological distress and compared it all to their ability to forgive others. Those who held on to their anger and resentment had the highest pain levels by far. Those who were able to forgive released a lot of their lower back pain (Carson et al. 2005).

Personal empowerment to heal comes with forgiveness. This research found that forgiveness doesn't simply reduce the level of anger. The act of forgiving is "significantly associated" with the use of fewer medications, less alcohol use, lower blood pressure and heart rate, and fewer overall physical symptoms of ill health (Lawler-Row et al. 2008).

Self-forgiveness is essential. Forgiving oneself for transgressions is an important part of the forgiveness process with positive implications for mental and physical health. A group of 141 study participants completed questionnaires about forgiveness and their health. Being able to forgive was associated with better overall health status, both mental and physical (Svalina and Webb 2012).

Motives for forgiveness are important. In two studies a team of researchers examined different motives for forgiveness in the

workplace involving coworkers who had offended the study participants. Five types of forgiving motives were identified: moral, religious, relational, apology, and lack of alternatives. "Individuals who
claimed to have forgiven because they believed they had no other
alternatives, or who forgave because they believed a higher power
(religious) required it, were more likely to report greater stress and
poorer health. Positive outcomes of forgiveness were discovered for
those employees who forgave because they believed it was the right
(moral) thing to do" (Cox et al. 2012).

Scientific research suggests that we can recover from the following ail-
ments much faster if we exercise forgiveness: alcoholism, anxiety, cancer,
cardiovascular disease, depression, drug addiction, high blood pressure,
hostility, pain, stress, and wounds. Caroline Myss, renowned health and
spirituality author, says that your biography becomes your biology. It's a
relief to know that these negative health conditions that were mostly self-
inflicted can be reversed.

I have been walking around with encyclopedic ignorance and guard-
ing it like it was priceless treasure. Maybe most people are this way; the
macho culture I grew up with sees acts of forgiveness as weakness. Once I
learned otherwise, I felt as if a heavy burden had been lifted from my heart.

Intimacy

About three or so weeks into my experiment I lost twenty-three pounds.
By the end of the fifth week, another nineteen pounds had dropped away.
The more weight I lost and the more I detoxed, the more emotional pain
I felt rumbling to the surface. Remorse about my father and brother came
up. Despair over my estrangement from my daughter, Lisa, and my ex-
wife, Mia, erupted to the surface. It seemed never-ending. So many layers
of the transformation onion needed peeling. I had over a half-century of
accumulated toxicity. I wasn't interested in an unfolding, organic process;
I wanted to get my shit together by Friday.

Every day the three amigos conducted a line of questioning about my life, digging in and getting beneath the surface. They were like New Age CSI interrogators. We might start out talking about the weather, and then suddenly one of them would ask a serious question. I knew what they were doing and why. I usually tried to deflect them with a lame attempt at humor.

"Frank, what do you say isn't the best about your life?" Ryland asked me on one occasion. In this instance he caught me off guard, and I didn't have a clever redirecting response. There was something painful hanging around at the forefront of my mind, and I couldn't ignore it.

"The thing I'd say that disturbs me the most about my life is my relationship with my daughter. Or lack thereof," I replied. "And my inability to find a way to fix it. To find a way to generate a conversation that is loving, a conversation that doesn't wind up in a place of accusation and insult and hurt."

Prior to this conversation I had just experienced a very difficult day. I lost my voice the night before after a difficult conversation with my daughter. I knew that I could have handled the interaction better than I had, but I always seemed to lose control, especially when I got the feeling that she didn't care whether we had a relationship or not. It was frustrating and powerful. (How much this discomfort and distress had to do with the detoxing and cleansing and everything else, I don't know. After ten years, I had suddenly stopped taking antidepressants, so there was a combination of contributing factors. I should not have done it this way, and I do not recommend it. If you want to change or stop your meds, *always* consult a competent medical practitioner first.)

When you have children with somebody, you are inextricably linked to that person for life, whether you like it or not. Mia and I had always had a turbulent relationship, and Mia would agree with that. We fought all the time. Some considered this behavior a reflection of passion. In retrospect, it was an indicator of madness. Turbulence between us was as common as the air; I could never figure out how to break that cycle, and I had grown weary of the contentious nature of our relationship.

There's something to be said about human beings and contact. I hadn't had genuine contact with a woman in a long time—except for a tango lesson during which I almost melted from the yearning for this woman who embraced me and led me around the room.

All of these swirling, rampaging emotions kept bringing me back to the realization that I would have to smooth the waters out with Mia in order to have a relationship with my daughter. If I could achieve that, I might even be ready for an intimate, loving relationship with a new partner. The three amigos, being the spokesmen for positive thinking, were very encouraging. I also knew from my 12 Step work and therapy that I had to look with unwavering focus at my side of the street.

Mia

I met Mia at a New York disco in 1977. She had a red carnation in her hair. Her skin was the color of warm dark honey. Completely mesmerized, I thought she was the most beautiful woman I had ever seen in my life. We exchanged numbers. When she called me, I thought, *Oh, my God! She actually called me back.* I couldn't believe it. We started talking and then going out. In the beginning I treated her like a piece of fine china; I was so captivated, I made no moves on her—just her presence was more than enough stimulation. Mind you, in those days a strong wind blowing my way would excite me. I finally realized how much I cared for her when I was alone in a darkroom, developing prints, and watching her image emerge in the tray. I knew I was in love.

It was a physical attraction that would last decades. Even after ten years of marriage, she could not get dressed or undressed in front of me without me chasing her around the house. Sometimes she would yell at me about something, and all I could think was *when she stops yelling at me, I'm going to fuck her.* That went on for a long time. Even after we got divorced, we had our interludes.

When we split up, Mia and I got involved in a stormy and bitter child custody dispute over our son, Nick, that lasted a year. Our daughter, Lisa, had taken sides with her mother and her mother's family. Now I wanted Mia and Lisa to see me as the person I had become rather than as the ghost of Christmas past. I wanted them to see that I had changed. I wanted my daughter to love me.

It was painful to think of my daughter holding resentment toward me. I wanted to redeem myself in her eyes. I was persistent in maintaining contact with her, always hoping we could get beyond the barrier between us. My shortcoming was that I had expectations when I called, while she wasn't ready to reconcile. A self-centered enterprise, resolution would help me feel better. Her continued rejection of me was becoming unbearable; she knew how I felt, and it seemed like she wanted to hurt me.

Both Mia and Lisa would indict me. It was devastating to hear them say things like, I didn't know how to raise Nick, and claimed that I provided him no discipline. I had been a terrible father to both of my children. I was a loser and a failure. My family's words had only served to reinforce my inner critic and the vitriol I was spewing on myself.

So how should I act when someone else refuses to forgive me? I could only start the healing where the pain made me feel most vulnerable. It was time to clear the mine field of all my past resentments and reactive behaviors, not just those surrounding the Catholic Church.

7

Love Is a Many-Splendored Thing, Week Six

Dear Mia,

I hope this letter finds you well and in good spirits.

We have known each other for nearly thirty years and raised two children.

Over the years I have, at times, responded with anger and resentment.

I want to apologize for all of the times that I was unreliable and emotionally irresponsible due to my drinking.

The anger that I held onto over the years was more empowering than to deal with how crushed I was when we divorced.

Even when we were in court, I looked across the aisle and wondered how love turns into litigation.

I began to believe that you never really loved me.

That feeling was too overwhelming.

Anger was a place of false power.

I would like you to consider the possibility of a relationship of trust and warmth.

A relationship where we can both be with our own children at the same time.

I apologize for my terrible behavior as I plunged head-first into the pit of addiction.

I have been clean and sober for seventeen years.

Many of the characteristics that I have demonstrated were triggered by alcohol.

That is not an excuse, it's just an explanation.

I invite you to consider that I am a different person.

You may have loved me, but I did not love myself.

As a result, I blamed you for my inability to feel loved by you.

I ask you to consider the possibility that we need not have a broken family.

What we could have is a mutual loving relationship with our children and release the broken record of hostilities.

I will always be grateful for you choosing me to be the dad of our beautiful Nick and Lisa.

Let us be an example of love and generosity and compassion.

I invite you and Lisa to come to San Francisco and be with who I am now.

Since this is an invitation, I will pay for the tickets.

Thank you for taking the time to read this letter.

I request that you respond as soon as you comfortably can so that I can arrange travel most convenient for you.

Frank

Earlier I described how one day at Café Gratitude I had been approached by and engaged in conversation with a woman I didn't know. In a fleeting exchange she said, "Love like you've never been hurt." That statement had been echoing across my neural canyons ever since. I couldn't even come close to imagining what that felt like, to love so fearlessly. The stranger's words had nestled in my heart.

My pattern with women was neurotic at best. If I met one I liked, I would try to make myself indispensable. Being a carpenter really came in handy. It's amazing what some women will do for a good carpenter. I was also a good cook, hustler, and problem-solver. I did it all not to be abandoned, which I always was, and to feel loved and needed, which, of course, I rarely did.

Throughout long-term and short-term relationships, it never occurred to me to be honest about who I was and what I was feeling. The thought of doing so blasted terror through my chest. *If you really knew me, you would never like me.* I was always abandoned, of course, though, because they were attracted to an impostor. One glimpse of the man behind the curtain, and whatever sparks had been died then and there. This pattern played out in nearly all my relationships, not just the romantic ones.

There was no denying that my behavior led to my daughter Lisa's emotional distance toward me. Reestablishing a relationship with her was the most important goal in my life, but in order to make inroads with Lisa, I had to make amends with Mia. At least, that's how I thought it should work.

Lisa had finished college and was working for a tech company in Sarasota, Florida, where Mia and her sister were also living. Mia agreed to come to San Francisco, but Lisa refused. Being with Mia was just the first hurdle on what would prove to be an emotional gauntlet.

Mia had never admitted or apologized for her side of what happened between us. I thought that if I accepted her lack of acknowledgment for her role, I would be able to let it all go. It had been a year or more since I had seen her, and she knew this visit was intended to be a reconciliation. The amigos saw this as a monumental potential breakthrough and were enthusiastic. It was to be a major turning point in my path to healing, and they wanted to witness the process.

The first day after her arrival we were on our best behavior. Yes, she stayed with me, and yes, we did sleep together.

The next day unfinished business started to brew between us. I wasn't prepared for the intensity of emotions that would culminate the eruption of Mount Vesuvius.

Under the Volcano

Ryland knocked on my door and entered, followed by the other two. The boys were anxious to see how I was doing. This time their mission was to meet Mia and satisfy their curiosity about how we would be treating each other.

Unfortunately, they had walked into the middle of a tempestuous argument about our thirteen-year-old son, Nick. A year earlier, I had sent Nick to Florida to spend time with his mom during summer break when she arbitrarily decided to keep him there. Nick was devastated and wanted to come back after having been with me for two years. I flew down to confront Mia and return Nick to California where he wanted to be. What ensued was a melodramatic cloak-and-dagger scene. While in Florida, Nick was under constant surveillance by someone in Mia's family. Nevertheless, Nick found a way to escape and made his way to my hotel room. We drove to the airport all the while anticipating an ambush by the police and terrified until we were up in the air. It was like the last scene in *Argo*.

When Mia and I started to talk about it, I had the unreasonable hope that she would be conciliatory if not apologetic. Instead she took what I interpreted to be an aggressive and self-righteous posture. That got me very pissed off. Enter the boys:

"Alright, Frank," Ryland announced. "It's the boys. What's been the experience?"

"My experience is that I'm still enraged," I exploded, pounding the counter with my fist. I could see from their facial expressions that the amigos were stunned and taken aback. I couldn't contain myself. As the boys sat down near Mia and me, their mouths were hanging open, and my rage was searing the air like a flamethrower.

"I am still so caught up in my anger toward my in-laws, and my daughter, and Mia. Part of my rage is that I feel like I can't do anything about it. I can't. And I fucking want to break my fucking brother-in-law's face! I want to smash my sister-in-law's face. I want to fucking hit all of them for letting this whole thing happen. To take away my ability to take care of my kids. To fucking do that to me and to not even question once whether or not what they were hearing or what they were assuming was true! And it's this gang of people that maintain this thing with my daughter. Because my daughter could not maintain this kind of feeling on her own."

"Whoa, whoa, whoa!" Mia snapped back at me.

"Shut the fuck up! I'm not interrupting you."

"You want the story to be—" Mia tried to continue.

"You want the story to be what? Your way? Fuck you!" I shouted.

"Until you see Lisa face to face and deal with her anger," Mia explained, "she's angry because of what she saw me going through, because you didn't see that! She saw it. I am trying to help you. And the way I can help you is to try to figure out what to do with the family over there and . . ."

Nothing Mia said could placate me. "Go tell Lisa that it was a fucked-up thing that everybody did! And maybe she'll start seeing. Maybe she'll start getting . . ."

"Do you think that?"

"Maybe."

"Don't you think that I have said things?"

"No!"

"To her?"

"No, no, I don't think that. I don't believe that anybody has said anything that remotely fucking resembles the truth to that kid! Not even remotely! Did anybody ever say to her that this was not right? No! Nobody ever said that. Because they can't. They haven't got the fucking balls! Nobody has the balls in that family to say, 'Hey, this was a wrong thing, let's deal with it!' We were right!"

"We have," Mia objected.

"Right! Yeah, fucking right! I've got to go. I'm so fucking crazy. I'm just so angry right now." I wanted to storm out of my own apartment, but the camera was rolling and the three amigos were staring at me, petrified.

"You did what you selfishly thought was right. You just cared about yourself, Frank. You didn't do it for Nick, because this whole fucking thing affected Nick too. What kind of psychological shit did you put him through? You didn't think about him! You thought about Frank!"

The worst of the storm had passed, though the air was still laden with the weight of broken hearts. Ryland was the first of the amigos to speak up. "You've come all this way," he said reassuringly.

"I feel like I didn't get anywhere. I know what you're saying. But at this moment I feel like I might as well have not gone anywhere. As miserable and as rageful and self-loathing as I feel right now, I might as well have still been a fucking dope fiend."

"Maybe you are bumping right up against what you need to bump up against," observed Conor, trying to be helpful.

"I'm bumping up to something, but you know what? Maybe I am, but I'm fucking tired of bumping up against shit, man. It's like I'm bumping up against shit all the time. I'm tired, man! I'm fucking tired of it. I'm tired of this rage. I'm tired of being pissed off. I'm stuck. I feel stuck."

"I want you to get this," interjected Ryland. "She's rooting for you and your daughter to have a relationship."

"Oh, I believe that," feeling defeated.

"She actually said it since we've been here," added Conor.

"I totally believe that."

"Acknowledge her for it!" said Ryland.

So I looked squarely at Mia and said, "I believe and I acknowledge that you want me and Lisa to have a good relationship. Unfortunately, I've been holding onto old stuff. Rather than acknowledge you for who you are now, I blame you for what happened before. So I apologize for that. I will try really hard to transcend that and be honest with you, not only because of you, but because it's just no good for me. I can feel it. Literally, it feels like it's tearing me up inside."

After my blowup I apologized to the three amigos. The guys were not used to being around explosive anger. I was ashamed of myself. Conor actually yelled at me during my rant, reprimanding me for losing my temper, but I was so out of control that what he said didn't register. Conor had been scared, not angry, and I could see the fear in his eyes. The depth of his fear startled me. I did not want to be the man I saw reflected in his face.

The amigos had wanted a nice clean love-fest; instead they wandered into a tectonic clash between a Puerto Rican and a Sicilian. My anger had little to do with the moment. Rage is archival. It may have been triggered by Mia, but she had nothing to do with the source of my apoplectic reaction. If it's hysterical, it's historical.

It was an expression of a deep wound from childhood—betrayal and cruelty; whatever traumas I had experienced as a kid, this incident triggered all of those things. My reaction to her was completely dispro-portionate to the incident. Having that tantrum in front of everyone was discouraging because I had thought the pain was behind me. I realized then that I had a lot more work to do. I wasn't as healed as I thought. I was still stuck in an old story, and my tirade was proof of it. I'd carved all sorts of new neural pathways, but there was more to excavate. Much more. My emotions were still triggered by the past.

When you let go of something you've identified with for years—whether it's a behavior, a thought, or a relationship—a feeling of emptiness arises. Unfortunately, we often prefer living with the unpleasant familiar rather than feel adrift in the emptiness that holds the promise—and the fear—of real change. Rage is an effective means of stagnation.

Transformation isn't linear. Life isn't linear. Sometimes it's two steps forward and one step backward. I felt like I took a huge step backward that day, but then . . . maybe not. Maybe in a strange sort of way this was a sign of progress.

Mia stayed for about a week. After the blowup, which was all docu-mented on camera, I was emotionally spent. I withdrew as my way of cop-ing. We were cautious and delicate with each other until she left.

My reconciliation work with Mia had no effect on Lisa. She had her own issues with me that remained unresolved. After Mia left I felt a mel-ancholy that blended with resignation. I let go of trying to sway Lisa and took a breather from the whole thing. Mia and I had intermittent con-versations for a while, mostly about Nick and Lisa. No more blowups oc-curred. I ended our communications before any acrimony could surge up and spiral out of control again.

Picking Up the Pieces

It was Conor's day to interact with me. We briefly talked about the blowup, using the Café Gratitude workbook. I felt lethargic, emotionally drained, and not fully engaged. I went through the motions of being responsive to Conor and his questions.

"Today is about love and acceptance," Conor began.

"Yeah, yeah." I knew what was coming like a train bearing down on me.

"Perfect after what you just went through. Now the thing is just getting you to see that."

"Yeah . . . yeah. I know. Resistance causes pain and lethargy. It is when we practice acceptance that new possibilities appear." I was repeating the expressions and words from the workbook without enthusiasm, just to get through the ritual. "Exploration. Acknowledge two events in life that you don't trust."

"Divinities," Conor reminded me.

"As Divinities of perfect expression," I continued reading. "Identify what it would take for you to bring love and acceptance to those events. Share them with your partner." I sat there in silence for a few moments. "I'm drawing a blank, man."

Patiently, Conor continued to work with me. "If you acknowledge that life as the divine was putting this in front of you for a reason—"

"It will be easier to swallow," I finished the thought.

"Right and there'd be more. As we were sitting there, she left and you just, like, flatlined, just . . . bbbrrrrrrrrrrrrrrrrrrrr," he murmured as his hand sliced horizontally. "And that's like the thing to trust. That interaction was divinity's perfect expression. It was the perfect thing to come up. Identify what it would take for you to bring love and acceptance to those events."

"What would it take?" I was in a fog of self-absorption.

"What would you have to let go of?" Conor clarified.

"I would have to let go of my doubts about who I am and what my motives are. Let go of what I think other people are thinking and let go of what other people tell me. And trust that fifty-four years on the planet did not render me a complete fucking moron."

"No. We're just on a forty-two-day path," Conor reminded me.

"Not all rosy."

"Not all rosy, but it's like this is the perfect thing to have come up. This is what you're after. This is the meat of what you want."

My blowup and embarrassing myself in front of everyone was the "perfect thing" to have come up? This was what I was after? The "meat" of what I wanted? I wasn't feeling any of that at the time, though intuitively I knew that Conor was on to something. Peeling off layers of the emotional onion isn't all about experiencing wine and roses. Personal transformation is often a messy process. Did I have what it takes to continue, or would I slide back into my old familiar toxic ways? Even I was in suspense about the outcome.

An Experiment Comes to an End

During those six weeks I wasn't just eating raw enchiladas, raw pizza, salads, zucchini noodles, or drinking the wheatgrass juice. I was hanging out, meeting people, and having animated, interesting conversations. I became a fixture at the café, and one of the perks was a steady stream of people to talk to, which offset my terrible loneliness.

I expanded my social network and met many warm and compassionate people. I didn't always know how to respond to expressions of kindness; as a result, I often responded inappropriately. I often reverted to flirting to avoid a deeper conversation. Afterward I would feel embarrassed by my behavior—they were simply offering kindness, and I made it into something else because of my own insecurities.

When issues are triggered, it's always a two-way street. My brand of humor and my background were different from what most millennial vegans were used to. They were cutting-edge, New Age, awareness types practicing their brand of political correctness. Their form of PC was new to me, so I occasionally rubbed someone the wrong way. It wasn't deliberate; I was a stranger in a strange land. When an Indian chef walks into your house, your kitchen is going to smell like curry. It takes a while for the olfactory glands to adjust. My Italian working-class street humor was abrasive to some. The three amigos were used to it and could handle it, but their coworkers always had a period of adjustment. Inviting me into their sphere became an experiment for all of us. The fact that I was such an anomaly in their world helped make the experiment interesting.

"I always feel judged by you," I told Matthew in one confrontation.

He replied that "everybody judges everybody, but it's the way you are with people, always with a wise-ass remark, making a joke, flirting. It has a negative impact on people."

I felt angry and hurt because he was looking at me through the lens of my past, and I wanted to be judged by my progress. He was another opportunity for me to practice radical forgiveness.

During those six weeks I was frequently called out on my self-deprecating humor. I'd say things like "well, what do I know, I'm just a dumb guinea from Brooklyn." I'd make jokes about my weight. Essentially, what I expressed as humor revealed a deeper truth. The three amigos and their family eventually made me agree that I would cease making any negative remarks about myself. That's when I noticed how much of my daily discourse was occupied by this unhealthy habit; I constantly put myself down. Armed with this new awareness, I was surprised by how much I did it and how I really saw myself. It made me sad. Why do I have the need to do that? I couldn't just say, "I won't do this anymore." All the self-deprecating humor was serving a purpose. I had to make room within for a bigger life.

I started questioning my chronic questioning. Maybe I do deserve to be loved. I carved new neural pathways by practicing restraint and not repeating all the critical things I was thinking about myself. With repetition I came to see another go-to place within myself. C. S. Lewis said that "the doors of Hell are locked on the inside." I was acting my way into a new way of thinking.

The end of my six-week experiment felt anticlimactic and uneventful. After so much time spent watching over me, the three amigos were grateful that it was over. It had taken up so much of their attention and time. They never expected me to last the entire forty-two days. We had shot around 120 hours of film. The movie needed editing, but no one had the experience or motivation to take it on. As time passed, so did my memory of the film. The footage went into a shoebox. We said our goodbyes and went our separate ways. I would still visit the restaurant, but the topic of the film never came up.

It ended in a whimper with no debrief or after-care. Therapists I talked to later on were appalled. "You can't just open a guy up and then leave him alone," one told me. In everyone's defense, it was an experiment, and we were all pilgrims in terra nuova. I tried to navigate the contours of my new life and fumbled and tripped. In the process, I woke the sleeping dragon, stopped going to 12 Step meetings, and forgot I was an addict. The resulting relapse brought me to death's door.

8

Relapse and Rebound

'Twas the night before rehab. . . .

I opened my eyes and saw faceless blue uniforms with silver badges over-running my dreary motel room, all talking loudly and moving quickly. One of the blue people leaned toward my bed, placed a black cuff over my bicep, and slipped a silver disc under the cuff. My eyes tried to follow the path of the stethoscope to the head it was attached to, but I kept falling back into my self-induced stupor.

The paramedic taking my blood pressure was speaking English, I felt sure of that, yet his words didn't compute. It sounded like gibberish. My eyes tried to fix on a frame of reference for what was happening, and I noticed two people at the foot of my bed staring down at me. Others in blue uniforms continued swirling around me, a frenzy of activity in the small room. It occurred to me that something serious was happening, and I was at the center.

One of the paramedics began examining an array of orange vials on the chipped Formica dresser. I noticed he didn't have a gun and felt relieved—at least they weren't cops. The labels all had my name on them anyway and had all been legally prescribed to me. I was an accident waiting to happen. The previous night I doubled my daily dose of prescription meds (which were already enough to put a small town to sleep): 100 mg of morphine sulphate, 100 mg of OxyContin, 150 mg of Norco, and a sprinkling of crushed Valium in the herbal tea I drank each night.

My friend Valerie had suggested I stay overnight in Alameda. It was a nondescript, anywhere-in-the-USA, no-tell, Motel 6 type of place. Distinguished only by the door number, all the rooms looked alike and were characterized by the smell of disinfectant, scratches on the dresser, and a remote control chained to the TV. The pool was unused. Later that night Valerie followed her intuition and came to check on me. She knocked on my door. Panic set in when she saw my car parked directly in front of the room but no answer from me. If she hadn't checked on me and made the 911 call, you wouldn't be reading these words right now. I would be dead.

"What year is it?" One of the voices demanded of me. I mumbled something. "What city are you in?" The voice bellowed at me. I mumbled something else, wondering all the while if I was stuck in a bad movie. "Who is the president?" My inquisitor demanded of me. It was clear I wasn't exactly Jeopardy game show material.

Maybe, as the saying goes, there are no accidents. I hadn't intentionally set out to commit suicide. On the contrary, I had checked into this dingy motel room to catch an early plane at the Oakland airport—I was headed to Hazelden treatment center in Oregon. I had developed a dependency on prescription drugs that I knew I had to break

The problem with consistent use of prescribed narcotics is that you never really know how high you are. Because the meds eliminated my anxiety, I actually thought I was normal and balanced most of the time. I was a functioning addict. My apartment was clean, my clothes ironed, my car well maintained, my papers handed in on time at grad school, but the prescription drugs were corroding my body, mind, and soul. My spirit was decaying as quickly as iron in salt water.

I stopped being diligent about the amount of prescription pills I was taking, and the dragon was alive and eternally hungry. At first, I tried to control it: When I woke up, I would count the amount of pills for the day. I kept a small pill box in the watch pocket of my jeans. If I didn't monitor the dose at the beginning of the day, I would lose track of how many pills I took. I was flirting with death, but my addict mind told me I was in control. My overdose was one layer of the onion. The deeper I peeled, the closer I came to my barnacled self. I realized how many more layers remained to be peeled back.

For six weeks I engaged in a radically different way of being. From living as a painfully lonely, reclusive fat guy, I had been thrust into the middle of a community and become the center of attention for sweet, idealistic youngsters. Life at that moment was getting incrementally brighter. Meanwhile, I was on hepatitis C medication and a slew of other drugs—I had been in carpentry for more than twenty years, which had been brutal to my body, going up and down those rickety ladders, using my leg to hold up walls; my left leg had been deteriorating and had become arthritic. Toward the end of my hep C treatment and as the six-week experiment got underway, my physician prescribed Vicodin of which I flushed the first bottle of sixty tablets down the toilet. I heard too many stories of relapses caused by this powerful painkiller. When I informed him I flushed the pills, my doctor got annoyed and said he would stop treating me unless I followed his protocol. Even though I told him about my fear of relapse, he didn't seem concerned and ordered me to "take them as prescribed." Despite my misgivings, I did as told.

By the fifth week of the experiment most of my doubts about taking the medications had disappeared. The entire program—being constantly around positive people, the daily affirmations, the cleansings and nutritious food—had really opened me up emotionally and physically. Although I started out taking the meds as prescribed, eventually I would say the words that precede every disaster: "Fuck it." In no time I had four doctors prescribing nuclear-powered pain killers. My kitchen counter looked like Walgreen's after a pharmaceutical delivery. All of it legal.

Around this time I stopped regularly attending 12 Step meetings, believing that the support I was getting through the experiment was enough—a mistake because the three amigos and their Café Gratitude community didn't grasp what it means to be an addict. Having a breakthrough and communicating with your ex-spouse or finally making that call to your dad or losing thirty pounds doesn't mean you understand the mind of a dope fiend. To be clear, I am not blaming my relapse on anyone or on any circumstance. Those six weeks would have been an ideal time to double up on attending meetings and talking to a sponsor or people who understood the scheming, deceptive, and manipulative face of addiction. I did neither. Instead, I followed doctor's orders and took another pill. The fantasy of every addict is that he can manage his own addiction. The pills were just another way not to feel. After seventeen years of sobriety, thousands of 12 Step meetings, hundreds of hours reading addiction literature, sponsoring, being sponsored, and absorbing more information about addiction than most physicians do, my addict mind told me that I could safely manage my narcotic intake.

On Christmas Eve 2005 I was closing down my apartment for a month. I put the guitars away from direct sunlight, vacuumed, threw out the trash and all perishable foods. I loaded up the car and drove to Alameda. It was to be the last night of my drug life.

When all of the paramedics left, I found myself feeling sicker than ever and totally beat up. My entire abdominal cavity was supremely sore. I later realized it hurt from all the retching. Even staying in bed was painful, but I remained there until it was time to leave for the airport.

Valerie drove me to the airport for my flight to the Hazelden in Oregon. I was so out of it that I had to be wheeled through the terminal. Except for my heartbeat, I felt dead. Once on the plane, I was surrounded by bubbly flight attendants wearing Santa Claus hats topped with white fuzzy balls and little bells. The plane was packed with traveling families. The scene was grotesquely surreal. I reached my moment of pitiful, incomprehensible demoralization. My bones felt fractured under the weight of unimaginable loneliness. My flight into Dante's ninth circle of Hell was ready for takeoff.

I was about to experience the longest twenty-eight days of my life.

To Tell the Truth

A nervous breakdown may be one of the most underrated forms of spiritual transformation—though I wouldn't recommend it without adult supervision. Hitting rock bottom *again* is a nightmare within a nightmare. Awakening to reality is like emerging from the cellar after the tornado has left. My head was filled with scavenger dogs roaming the wreckage, glaring menacingly, reminders of dark deeds long forgotten. In this tortured psychic state, I manufactured the delusion that all would be normal and manageable by the end of twenty-eight days, a pathetic attempt at self-soothing. In reality it would be nearly a year before the neurochemistry, biochemistry, and my attitude normalized.

For forty-two days I was committed to staying on a healthy path with the three amigos—I had opened my own emotional cookie jar. Despite all the work I'd done and all the support provided me, I let myself drift back into the pit of addiction. I stepped away from my pals at Café Gratitude, and I stepped away from the 12 Step program. I'd fallen off my new positive bandwagon and climbed onto an old, familiar one. I was like memory plastic: I could be molded into any shape, but, if exposed to enough heat, I would revert back to my original form.

Relapse is a terrible experience. It creates heartache and wreckage in other people's lives, not to mention the potentially lethal outcome for the addict. Addiction corrodes the body and soul. Like many addicts, I made up my own rules as I went along and began to believe my own bullshit. There are none so blind as those who will not see.

I had scheduled rehab for December 24 to January 21, between the fall and spring semesters. Hazelden in Springbrook, Oregon, specializes in treating people in the medical profession. My dorm was occupied by general practitioners, doctors, anesthesiologists, surgeons, and pharmacists. These were high-profile, accomplished addicts uncovering, discovering, and discarding aspects of who they were or thought they were. Addiction is the great equalizer. We may have arrived in different ships, but we were all in the same boat now.

Soon after arriving we did a group exercise in which we each chronologically listed our addictions from the beginning. Some started with candy, others with cigarettes. I churned out three pages of behaviors; it was ego-deflating to sit there and recite my legacy of addictions to everyone in the circle. The experience served to reveal that I was just another garden-variety alcoholic/drug addict. The only difference between a high bottom and low bottom is a bank account.

For most of my life I conformed to whatever gained the most acceptance. As a kid, I developed mechanisms to avoid physical pain. Some worked, some didn't. I began to perceive the world as conspiratorial and hostile. Every authority figure in my life was punitive. It's not like I was beaten and tortured all the time, but just enough to cloud every decision and almost every action I took. I came to see the world as a courtroom, and my quest was to prove my innocence.

Before that moment in rehab, it never occurred to me to tell the truth. Why would I when telling the truth usually caused some kind of pain? As a child, the people who encouraged me to be honest would say, "If you tell the truth, you'll have nothing to worry about." What a crock of shit. When I said, "Well, Sister, if that were true, why would we need lawyers?" she responded with a lightning-quick slap to my young face. The reality was that in my world it was dangerous to reveal my feelings or ideas. Doing so often resulted in ridicule or retribution. What comes up in rehab is just about everything. Whether sharing in a group setting, conferring with a counselor, or journaling, it's a verbal and mental regurgitation of your entire life. Mine started with my family upbringing.

Passion and Violence Share the Same Coin

Protestants have drama. Italians have opera. I often felt like I was living in a perpetual performance of Pagliacci. We were a Catholic, working-class, Italian-American family in Brooklyn. There were no white picket fences or fields of green. My early life was a cross among *On the Waterfront*, *Blackboard Jungle*, and *Goodfellas*—many of my neighbors were low-level mafia with a sprinkling of middle management.

As a young kid I had the heart of a poet, but in order to survive I had to learn how to either fight or talk fast. I was the eldest of four, three of whom got seriously into drugs—two slayed the dragon, and one became the sacrificial lamb. My younger sister, Patricia, died in her early thirties after a life of dancing with the devil only to be consumed by the flames. She left seven of her own children whom we know of, strewn out into the world, unmoored and unloved. There are no words to describe the incalculable magnitude of that tragedy. I defer to my brother Angelo, who summed up our family this way: "primarily, it ended up the way it did because we had no good guides. We had no fucking good guides."

The "guides" we *did* have instilled in me a huge fear of the Almighty, which came in two forms: the Church and my father. The nuns *found personal solace by inflicting cruelty upon children*. They taught me to believe that I was born with original sin. Upon learning this, at the tender age of six, I surmised that I was already in trouble for something I didn't do. Mahatma Gandhi said: "I like your Christ, I do not like your Christians. Your Christians are so unlike your Christ." My feelings exactly.

My father was a decent guy trapped in the body of an angry longshoreman. He was born in Palermo in 1911. During the 1920s Sicily was not roaring with anything but poverty. Both of my dad's parents died when he was a boy. He was shuttled around from aunt to uncle or whoever could afford him. When he was a teenager, he was diagnosed with a terminal illness (I never learned the nature of it), and since he thought he was going to die, Pappa decided to see America before the end and stowed away on a ship bound west.

In those days ships still used sails along with engines. It took twenty-five days to reach Norfolk, Virginia. During the crossing he puked every day. He was absolutely positive that his lethal illness had been expelled into the ocean. My father was arrested upon arrival, and, since he couldn't read or write English, a guy in his jail cell helped him fill out some documents. One of the questions had to do with political affiliations. His helpful cellmate checked the Communist box. That hair-thin stroke of ink would haunt my father for years to come.

Ironically, my father was apolitical. During the war he would sell guns to the Arabs and dynamite to the Jews. For him, it was always about survival. He witnessed the madness of war, fascism, Nazis, and the reign of Mussolini.

My father's demons were real and had the power to kill with impunity.

83

He was prone to violent rages that he often took out on me. Not feeling the necessity to change his situation, his idea of personal transformation was going from rags to riches—something he never did. Reinvention was not in his vocabulary. His most heart-felt piece of advice to me: "Don't ever become a pimp or a fag, or I'll kill you."

As a result, my inner life was a battle ground of conflict and contradiction. I became a persistent seeker of God and a fan of oblivion. I was filled with fear, anxiety, anger, and self-loathing. I also tried to kiss this earthly plain goodbye twice—or three times if you count the accidental overdose. Each time, I was surprisingly unsuccessful at negotiating my own demise. Addiction is suicide on the installment plan.

My parents didn't drink or do drugs. If they had, their behavior would have made more sense. My father was mercurial. One day he would be happy, laughing, telling stories about his years in the Italian Navy and Merchant Marines. At the height of his good mood he'd say, "Tomorrow we'll go buy a bike." The next day he would get angry if I brought it up. If I brought it up more than once, he would ridicule the way I asked him and then he'd hit me. I was never really sure how to act. None of this excuses my bad behavior; at the same time I was led to believe that being truthful was dangerous. In later years, this fear of being honest would manifest in a lack of integrity in my relationships with romance and finance.

In order to continue the long road to recovery, I had to learn what my truth was. I was dismayed to discover that the truth changes and that reality is fundamentally difficult to grasp. Interestingly, alcoholics and addicts, people who live to be stoned, believe they have a firm grip on reality. I learned that most people have a spectacularly narrow view of the here and now. I had tried to live my parent's truth, the Vatican's truth, the American truth, and perceived truth fueled by drugs and booze. Now I had to start all over and uncover my truth, an endeavor that will take me to my last breath.

Miracles championed by the Catholic Church sounded great to me. But I found an easier route to Divinity: drugs. Drugs helped me touch the Divine and gave me a sacred sense of relief. The first time I ever got loaded I said to myself, "Holy shit, *this* is how you get through life. *This* is how you do it." But that euphoria wore off. I thought I was supposed to feel like Superman. Instead, I ended up feeling like a loser.

During rehab, images of my life flickered by like images in a flip book. I flirted with the law, dope, and with booze. In the '60s amphetamines became my Lolita. I surrendered my soul to speed the way Humbert surrendered his to Lolita/Dolores. I kept the company of mortal sinners and ragged saints who came in the form of drifters, dopers, trust fund sociopaths, hippies, hookers, accidental Buddhas, criminals, and cons. Together we engaged in assorted acts of low- and high-brow defiance, some of which involved guns and other unpleasant objects. My life became a rhapsody of depression and despair. This unhappy state led to my first suicide attempt and to the psychiatric ward of Kings County Hospital. It takes angels to conquer demons. My better angels were asleep in the poppy fields. They kept sleeping when I tried to kill myself again two years later.

I was only twenty-seven years old, but when I closed my eyes, I could smell my own death. I took a cocktail of pills, wine, and methadone and jumped onto the subway tracks in New York City. I remember how the glimmer of the train's lights got brighter as the train curved toward the station and how the squeal of racing steel reached a crescendo. I was ready to meet my maker and experience the absolute oblivion that had always beckoned at the fringes of my consciousness. Instead, a gust of frigid wind blew as the roar diminished behind me. I lay there, dumbfounded. The subway echoed with the sound of receding metal. I was on the wrong track.

I spent most of the 1980s earning my bread and butter as a carpenter. I was also intermittently employed as a New York City cab driver, scrap metal hauler, dishwasher, census taker, warehouse stock boy, mail boy, ditch digger, club bouncer, general contractor, actor, and radio announcer. I was also a pot smoker, an alcoholic, a junkie, a speed freak, a cocaine aficionado, an avid reader, a father, a husband, a good guy, and a bad guy.

In 1987, shortly after Mia had our second child, Nick, I moved our family to Arlington, Virginia to get closer to nature and as far away from drugs and alcohol as possible. That didn't work. Wherever you go, there you are. As that decade came to a close, I was either drunk or hungover. I became the person I swore I'd never be. In 1989 the Berlin Wall fell apart and so did my life. I joined a 12 Step program and vowed to become sober once and for all. I credit that program with saving my life.

Like many in the recovery tribe, my relationships were almost always perverse, delusional, grandiose, dishonest, and fear-based. When I got sober, my daughter was eight and my son was two. Mia and I had been married for over ten years. Long ago we stopped pretending that any kindness remained between us. All our romantic gestures had bled to death. On our tenth anniversary Mia gave me a card that made a play on an old Timex watch commercial. The picture on the card was a room full of broken or destroyed household objects, furniture appliances, pictures, and papers strewn about. In the middle of the debris was a crumpled marriage license with the caption, "Takes a licking, but keeps on ticking." My insides felt like the face of that card. I was destroyed, and I had done it with my own hands.

During the divorce process in 1991, on a cold February evening, I found myself walking around Georgetown in Washington, DC, feeling miserable and sorry for myself. Everything was closed. The city was cold, empty, and dark. The street lights and gusts of wind amplified the dreary desolation. I came upon a place that happened to be open. The Yes! Bookshop.

It was warm and calm inside. The only person in the store was the clerk, who was Hindu and dressed in white with a white turban. I perused the books: *The Seat of the Soul, Care of the Soul,* hundreds of titles regarding spiritual growth and happiness. Rather than comfort me, the titles triggered a deep sadness. I felt like I had missed every boat I should have sailed on. I looked up at my turbaned friend and said, "You know, man, I could have really used this information when I was in my twenties."

"Yes," he said.

"But this material would've bored me to death. I could never have read through this stuff."

He paused, looked at me like the Cheshire Cat, and said, "That is how the information protects itself from you."

I walked into that February postmortem chill like a child lost in the woods. My soul was as frozen as the ice on the banks of the Potomac River. I used to think my problem was addiction. When I got sober, I was horrified to discover the problem was much worse. The problem was me.

A Day at a Time

If 12 Step programs were a branch of the military, some people would have earned Purple Hearts and Silver Stars. The way certain individuals maintain grace and dignity in the face of serious tragedies continues to inspire me. I have met people whose children have died unexpectedly, as well as people who faced financial ruin and fatal illness. Not only did these individuals remain sober, they maintained their dignity and self-respect. They are my heroes. These were broken and shattered men and women who now serve as examples of spiritual nobility. I thrive in the presence of energy like this. I want to hang out with these people in the afterlife.

Doctors, psychiatrists, social workers, psychologists, cops, courts, and religions have all made attempts to deal with addiction with dismal results. My sobriety was accomplished through one addict talking to another. Therapy is wonderful for the addict working the program, but therapists and psychiatrists have little or no effect on someone in the midst of addiction. In the end, people who transcended the heart of darkness helped me toward the light. It took angels with broken wings to illuminate a path toward my redemption.

Today nearly everybody knows something about rehab, or think they do. Famous people write about their treatment experience (rock stars, movie stars, lawyers, doctors). I have nothing new, profound, or enlightening to share on the subject. I only have my experience, sans pontification or evangelizing. I only know what works and doesn't work for me. Even with that understanding, I have consultations with my mentor and friends to prevent a collision with delusional thinking.

When I went to my first 12 Step meeting in 1989, I was at a complete loss as to how it could possibly work. People were milling around, talking and laughing; others were serious and quiet. In those days people still smoked at meetings—I mean they really smoked. The room was small with no windows and a low, acoustic, once-white tile ceiling that changed into a putrid excuse for yellow. I was amazed to see so much coffee consumed so quickly. I noticed that anxiety was frequently mentioned during the meeting. My first thought was maybe they should stop drinking so much fucking coffee. I surmised these people were not all too swift—this coming from a guy still experiencing the remnants of hangover from the day before.

I was afraid to raise my hand and share at that first meeting because I didn't know the protocol. People might tell me to shut up because I wasn't a member. Toward the end the speaker asked, "Are there any burning desires?" This sounded like safe harbor to me, so I raised my hand and said, "My name is Frank, I'm an alcoholic. I need help, but I don't know what to do." When the meeting ended, I was immediately surrounded by angels disguised as construction workers, real estate agents, salesmen, lawyers, and all those in between. All of them sober alcoholics and dope fiends.

That night was the end and the beginning. I was toxic with booze and cocaine and had no idea of what was going on. Bob was the first guy who spoke to me. He was a contractor building a deck in Arlington and offered me a job paying scale wages. He was kind and generous because he was getting less than his money's worth with me. It was hard for me to focus. My perspiration was like Alien's blood—I was afraid that my sweat would set the wood on fire. My job was to cut lumber, and I prayed the measurements he asked for would be either on the inch or half-inch. If he started calling out fractions, I would have a hard time seeing the tape. At one point, I accidentally shot my hand with a nail gun. Bob never fired me.

I thought this guy hired me because he had incurred an enormous karmic debt, and employing me would free him from his burden. In any case, I stayed sober long enough to keep staying sober. I was grateful for the job and his kindness. I felt that the least I could do for *these people* was not get loaded. That frame of mind will not sustain sobriety in the long run, but it did that day and that's what mattered. In the beginning, there are many things that keep people coming back to meetings. It doesn't matter what the reason as long as you don't pick up a drink or a drug that day.

"I'll never have fun again." I thought that was the price I would pay for sobriety. I was scared and depressed about my life dissolving into noth-ingness. Not that I was having any fun toward the end. I was miserable, and that's why I cleaned up. It is by circumstance rather than virtue that I wound up in recovery. Nevertheless, I thought I was waving goodbye to excitement from the back of a train—every click-clack of the steel wheels pulling me farther away from any pleasure. That belief keeps a lot of peo-ple from coming into recovery. They are still looking for that first high. I spent twenty-five years chasing 1968. When I was drinking and using, I thought I was living fully, but I was never fully present. There was a time when I wanted to learn to fly. Instead of taking lessons, I got stoned with a pilot I met at Arturo's, a bar in Greenwich Village. After several vodkas, a few lines, and a night full of excited banter, my flying experience was com-plete and a real airplane seemed insignificant. Booze and drugs robbed me of my best intentions.

A group of us got sober at the same time. We were like a freshman class, or a little tribe of gypsies lost and found at the same time. Something mystical occurs when groups like this band together. We were lost at sea, but together we ceased going further adrift. I was sharing a two-bedroom apartment in southwest DC with a sober fellow traveler when I decided to throw a party. I always liked parties. I was pretty broke at the time, but for about twenty bucks I could buy enough pasta and sauce and grated cheese for fifteen people. Even though I was sure no one would come, I invited a bunch of my fellow crazies for Saturday night spaghetti dinner. Who did I think I was that people would come to my house to be sober and still have a good time? I was wrong. They all showed up, and they stayed late.

We did this often during the winter months of my early sobriety. My son was two years old; my daughter was eight. The shy people played with my kids all night. Nick and Lisa had no idea how crazy their playmates were but didn't care either. Maybe sharing coloring books with the kids kept the scorpions in these addicts' heads at bay. The kids thoroughly en-joyed coloring with the asylum inmates, two of whom were totally deaf.

My living room became a refugee camp full of frightened souls holding onto each other amidst a smattering of Diet Cokes and spaghetti-stained paper plates. In retrospect, these events helped me get by when my brain was full of broken glass. As I began to calm down, I took pleasure in going to the movies, riding a bike, roller-skating, and spending time with my kids at petting zoos or pumpkin patches. Living sober enabled me to expand my life and start collecting new memories, feelings, and sensations. Memories I could reflect on when times were not so bright. Memories that would get me back to the present.

My coping skills were sophomoric at best. I eventually found that hanging out with positive people helped me see a new way of being. If you are determined to be miserable, chances are you will achieve a resounding success. On the other hand, if you let yourself have fun, you usually do. (If you aren't sure about what you consider fun, do some research. There are many books about ways to get high without drugs. These books cover activities from astral traveling to yoga and everything in between. Or just search "highs without drugs" in your internet search engine, and see what comes up.) Take a risk, try something different. Look for new sensations. Drugs may briefly exhilarate the senses, but, ultimately, they deaden everything. Positive new sensations sharpen the mind and free the spirit. Good memories are like investments. Diversify your portfolio.

As an addict, my idea of normal is to feel good all the time. I came into recovery with underdeveloped coping skills. I couldn't distinguish one feeling from another. My emotional landscape was like different vapors in one container. I was afraid of everything. When people were kind to me, I was uncomfortable. When people were short with me, I was uncomfortable. One minute at a time I began settling into my own skin.

When I was getting high, my biggest insecurity was running out of booze and drugs. When I got sober, I was insecure about running out of everything. I got in touch with the "never enough syndrome" in a different light. No matter how much love I received, I felt unloved. If I didn't have a job, I was afraid of not getting a job. If I had a good job, I was afraid of losing that job or I was resentful that I wasn't being recognized. I was living with deprivation mentality in the extreme. My mind was encumbered with thoughts like, "If she would only do this or that, everything would be okay." Or, "as soon as I get my shit together, everything will fall into place." I was on the cusp of an epiphany. It's *all* an inside job; as Carl Jung says, "It is amazing what people will do to avoid looking into their own soul."

My sense of "lack" is never current as its genesis resides in my archival past. I would have to practice neuro-transfiguration to live comfortably in the present. As an addict, I was reluctant to face my fears. Rather than look inside, I ran into the arms of my heroin addiction. Getting loaded was a long, slow, corrosive experience. Feelings of emptiness, of never having enough, were what drove the eternally hungry beast that was devouring my spirit. My way of coping was to use every conceivable manner of substance, money, drugs, food, reckless behavior, and alcohol to near lethal excess. It was never enough to fill the perceived void. I lived in the illusion of the black hole. In reality the soul is complete and whole just the way it is. The emptiness is all in my head.

Addiction is something that I do repeatedly that's contrary to my best interests—and I *know* it is contrary to my best interests. By definition, it's something I can't stop doing irrespective of the consequences. In that light, we're all addicts to one degree or another about something. Addiction is a cunning beast and a spiritual malaise that manifests in all sorts of things: food, drugs, alcohol, work, sex, shopping, hoarding. It's also an attachment to behaviors like lying and stealing and to feelings of anxiety, fear, depression, self-deprecation, rage, and anger. (If you want to know more about all of that, read several of Christopher Kennedy Lawford's books including *Recover to Live: Kick Any Habit, Manage Any Addiction*, and *What Addicts Know: 10 Lessons from Recovery to Benefit Everyone*.)

In my travels touring with the film, I have been stunned by the staggering number of people, addicts and non-addicts, suffering from the same joy-shattering malady: fear. Fear of not being loved. Fear of not being enough. Buried somewhere in the brain is the loop that repeats: *If you really knew me, you would never love me*. You don't have to be an addict or an alcoholic to have that tape playing in your head.

Those unfamiliar with addiction—including many therapists and doctors—don't realize that abstaining from your drug of choice (including food) without altering your consciousness will not free you from the root of your problem.

Buddhists talk about "ego clinging," which Pema Chodron describes as being attached to a fixed identity. "When things fall apart," she writes, "you feel as if your whole world is crumbling. But actually it's your fixed identity that's crumbling" (2012, 8). That is supposed to be cause for celebration—maybe so. I don't know about you, but the process of ego-shattering has never compelled me to kick up my heels and dance.

Overcoming the compulsion to abuse food or drugs is only the first of the hurdles. A quote often misattributed to Mark Twain goes, "It's easy to quit smoking. I've done it a thousand times." The causes and conditions that precipitated the abuse is where healing needs to be focused. Abusing food, drugs, sex, or whatever is an adaptive behavior by the addict because reality is unbearable. The voice that tells us to overindulge in drink or drug or food or sex is the same voice that afterward tells us what losers we are for abusing ourselves after we pick up.

It was only when the pain of my addict life became greater than my fear of my inner life that I was able to stop using and begin living clean and sober one day at a time. That was true the first time I got sober, and it was doubly true the second time around.

The Silver Lining

In rehab, I felt so sad and separate. I thought I would never laugh again. I was sure that I had done irreparable harm to myself. Minutes in rehab felt like years. The narcotic withdrawal involved extreme pain and discomfort. And I wasn't sleeping or eating. It all felt like a bad dream and another failed attempt at changing my life. It was like someone hitting me over the head with a hammer while I was trying to listen to music.

One morning while waiting for a group session to begin I was day-dreaming about my son and daughter. They were walking down the street. In the fantasy someone asked Lisa "How's your dad?" and Lisa says, "My dad is dead."

"How did he die?" she was asked.

"No one knows if it was a suicide or an accidental overdose," she replied.

In a flash I felt the pure, unadulterated selfishness of my behavior. The thought that I would leave this as a legacy to my kids. For the first time I felt the depth of that selfishness that defined my addiction.

It was a free fall into a mine shaft—a place every recovering addict knows. In a split second the burden and madness of my addiction came crashing down on me. Images of betrayal, neglect, cruelty, and stupidity flashed like a slide show at machine-gun speed. The lies and pain I caused were so close. I felt the bone-splintering weight of my desperation. My head collapsed in my hand. I cried like I'd never cried before. I felt like I was expelling ancient evil from my lower intestine.

I tried to catch my breath. I was turned inside out. For a time, I no longer existed. I was reduced to a blob of ectoplasm taking up space on the floor. I wept for them, and I wept for myself. I saw the blood and guts of my reality. It was ego crushing. It was emotionally devastating. It was my moment of clarity.

There's only one thing more painful than "I fucked up" and that's "I fucked up—*again*." There are no lessons more redemptive and powerful than the ones you learn when you're on your knees. Things sometimes have to fall apart before they can come together again.

The following days were extremely dark. My head was a death camp of my own design. I was to endure the three days in the tomb. The resurrection was nowhere in sight. Rebirth is a tidy term. The birthing experience is anything but. Transformation is messy, dramatic, frightening, and painful. The outcome is unpredictable. Faith is being ok with not knowing.

I had to create a shift in my life but I lacked the vision of what change looked like. It was certain that I either change or die. Thankfully, I can't see the future. If I'd had any idea what I was about to undergo, I'm sure I would have put it off. Never in my wildest imagination did I see myself eating raw food for forty-two days while taking directions from a bunch of twenty-somethings, much less that I would relapse after seventeen years of sobriety and then end up in rehab. No way! It was just inconceivable.

Only three friends knew I was in rehab. I was too ashamed to tell anyone else, especially my kids. While in session with the family counselor she observed that no one—not a friend, not a family member—had visited me since I arrived there.

"What about your family?"

"I haven't told anyone," I replied. "I feel that telling my daughter will destroy my relationship with her forever. I just hinted to her that I would be away."

"If you don't come clean with your relationships, you will never stay clean," she was kind but firm. Even in my acute withdrawal state, I knew she was telling the truth. Through all the cacophony and stupor clouding my mind, truth found a way through.

"Okay, I will call her."

The counselor suggested I commit to a day and time. I said a little prayer before making the phone call—the serenity prayer. I also prayed for the right words to say. I've come to believe that prayer is calling forth the light within.

We weren't allowed cell phones in rehab, so I went to a phone booth in the hall. After a few pleasantries I said, "There is something I need to tell you. Right now I am in rehab. I was afraid to tell you I got hooked on drugs again."

I expected her to condemn me as a loser; instead there was a long pause: "Gee, Dad, I thought you went to Mexico to get an exotic cancer treatment or something."

Once again my nondisclosing, untruthful behavior hurt someone. I lied for the sake of making an impression, while all this time she thought I was dying. I was doing the exact opposite of anything noble. Dishonesty is an act of emotional violence rooted in cowardice.

That conversation with Lisa broke the ice. It was pivotal. I told her, "I love you very much, and I want to resolve everything between us."

When I came out of rehab, I was still trembling. The prescription narcotics had taken their toll. At home I was agoraphobic for the first time in my life—leaving the house took such effort that I was exhausted by the time I arrived at my destination. I had started entering the stage of addiction withdrawal referred to as post-acute withdrawal syndrome. My counselors had told me exercise would relieve the paralytic anxiety I was feeling. The problem was that every time my heart rate accelerated even a little, I would be thrown into a panic attack or intensified anxiety. I was reaping the rewards of my decision to resume a way of dealing with life that went nowhere. My addict mind told me that I could handle it, but the addict mind can rationalize anything.

One of the most startling things I ever heard at a 12 Step meeting was said by a young woman: "Addiction is the only thing I know that is stronger than a mother's love." She told how she would drive to score drugs with her very young children and sometimes leave them in the car while she went to visit her connection. The obsession to use dominates the entire hard drive. When craving runs the show, everything else is secondary at best. I would wake up in terrible anxiety questioning the value of my life, so I made a practice of reading sections from *A Course in Miracles* and then meditating. If I was still in a bad place, I'd call someone. I engage in this practice to this day. Since I had perpetuated my drug life by surrounding myself with people who got high, I began to stay clean and sober by surrounding myself with people who were living sober and who believed in healing their lives. We addicts take turns talking each other off the ledge. Someone talks me off the ledge on Monday. I may do the same for someone on Friday. Thank God we're not all fucked up on the same day. Bad weather and passing thunderstorms don't have to be a permanent weather pattern.

Three months after I got out of rehab my daughter flew to San Francisco and stayed with me for a week. We did the tourist thing since she had never been to the city before. I took her to Fisherman's Wharf, Twin Peaks, Alcatraz, the beach, and Sausalito. It was the best time I had with her since she was a little girl.

As I reflect on rehab and the six weeks of my experiment with the boys, I see all of the parts of my life that these experiences have touched— places I was numb to, places I couldn't see or feel, and now I can. The experience in rehab was like walking through a nightmare in a straitjacket. When I checked out, a few of the guys wrote notes and cards about how I had helped them. I had no memory of doing so. I had no awareness of my impact on other people.

My initial wish was to fall in love one more time before I die. What I realize now is that the person I needed to fall in love with all along was me. Finding self-love is a process. It is also a gift. It serves as a positive foundation for a relationship with my daughter and with people in general. Having my daughter, Lisa, back in my life was the most wonderful gift of all.

By taking contrary action to my old ways, I began to carve new neural pathways. I created another go-to place for an impulse to land. It's not a fail-safe system—I have to practice curbing my impulses—but it gets better with time. Self-transformation isn't a linear process. Even the Dalai Lama has his bad days . . . or so I'm told.

9

Validation and Vindication

A year passed since rehab, and in that time I remained clean and sober, completed two semesters of graduate school at San Francisco State University, and developed new friendships. Unfortunately, I gained more weight than I lost during the six weeks with the three amigos. I was back to my old ways of frequenting Indian buffet restaurants. The drugs had left my system, and food was taking their place. I rearranged the deck furniture on the Titanic. I was also engaging in self-deprecating humor and negative attitudes again.

One day after a 12 Step meeting I was talking to a few friends, telling stories and making jokes at my own expense. After everyone dispersed, my friend Robert Keehan said, "I never let anybody put my friends down. When you say something bad about yourself, it's like someone insulting my friend. I don't like it, man. It feels bad to me."

I felt sad, embarrassed, and exposed. His statement took the wind out of me. It so happened that Robert had two master's degrees, one was in health science. He was also an amateur athlete. Robert said he could help me lose twenty pounds in a month if I followed his directions to the letter. That included being respectful to myself. I surrendered to the unknown again. The most important lessons I've learned in life were a result of challenging a fear or venturing into the unknown. It is in the heart of uncertainty that courage reveals itself.

My journey to fitness with Robert lasted over a year. He became my coach, guide, and my good friend. Going to the gym with him was purgatory in the beginning. Everyone looked thinner, more energetic, and happier than I could ever be. On the stationary bike I was exhausted and gasping after five minutes. I felt like a loser in the midst of winners, but I kept going back, day after day, sometimes twice a day. Upon reflection, I recognized a resilience I never acknowledged. I thought about the six-week Café Gratitude experiment, drug rehab, the subsequent year of recovery, the rigors of grad school, and therapy. Just as I made myself accountable to all of the above, I made myself accountable to Robert. I was resuscitating a dormant heart.

I spent an hour at the gym five times a week. The wonderful thing about working out is that in the beginning the results are dramatic. I completely eliminated all carbohydrates and sugar for the first year. During that time I ate a primarily plant-based diet. I rode the bike and did circuit weight training. By the time I reached my desired weight I went through five wardrobes. Robert was my accountability partner. He was there for me until I was there for myself.

Still weighing heavily on my heart were the results of all my life choices. I knew that if I let my shame dictate my next move, I would walk out of that gym and never come back. So I kept going back to challenge my fear and doubt. While working with Robert I let go of 120 pounds. The disciplined practice I developed with him paid off in unanticipated ways. Not in the least of which is a lifelong friendship.

For as long as I can remember I wanted to skydive. After watching *The Bucket List* with Jack Nicholson and Morgan Freeman I was even more determined. Coincidentally, I had a friend who was a skydiving pro. She had jumped 199 times and was going for number 200. When I told her I was interested in taking the plunge, she promised to do her milestone jump with me. Even though I had been eating intelligently and working out regularly, I still had more work to do.

When I phoned the skydiving facility to find out the particulars, they asked me a bunch of questions and all was going well until this one: "How much do you weigh?"

"Around 225."

"Sir, our equipment is certified for a maximum of 200 pounds."

You can't just think your way out of attachments or negative feelings. I certainly couldn't. I had to act in a new way of thinking. Going to a gym consistently and eating intelligently were commitments to my well-being, especially in those dark moments when I wanted to give up. After another month of diligent exercise I lost another twenty-five pounds. I was shocked and inspired by what I had accomplished.

There should be a fund established for anyone having a problem with faith in a higher power. This fund would pay for free skydives. When the plane door opens at 18,000 feet, the first thing you say is, "Oh, God!" In early November 2009, well before the deadline Robert and I had established, my friends Maritza and Bruce and I went off to skydive. This time, the feeling of free fall was exhilarating and nothing like tumbling down a mine shaft headed toward rock bottom. I had another motivation to hurl myself out of a perfectly good airplane. If I could face the terror of jumping out at 18,000 feet, I could draw on that moment to face whatever else in life frightened me. In other words, I thought skydiving would enhance my courage overall. Skydiving takes courage; the caveat is that the testicular fortitude necessary to expel oneself into the air is not transferable to ground use. I felt good about facing my fear and jumping. But I had to remind myself once again that there is no magic bullet or miraculous shortcut to self-transformation or spiritual growth. There are setbacks on the journey, just as walking across hot coals doesn't help you walk through the flames in your head.

The guy running with the ball always risks being tackled.

May I Be Frank Goes on the Road

The documentary about the experiment wasn't released until three years after I completed drug rehab and four years after filming. I had forgotten about it. It all seemed like a dream. The film is a testament to idealism—it's a miracle that it got finished. The youthful naiveté on the part of the boys and their film editor was a wonderful energy; they didn't concern themselves with the how and the why. I was reintroduced to the intoxicating notion of idealism, the place where possibilities shine brightly, a place I had last known in the 1960s.

Editing the movie was a labor of love for director Gregg Marks. Before Gregg, the film consisted of 140+ hours of unedited tapes in a shoebox. His vision of the narrative, along with the incredible support of producer Jeff Lamont and many others, made the completion of the film possible.

While touring with the film, I met many extraordinary people. In Boulder, Colorado, my host informed me that a local colon hydrotherapist had offered me a free session the morning after a screening. I set out with Gregg to find our new friend and irrigation specialist at a business park complex. I always get lost in these places. From a distance I saw a tall lanky guy with a long gray ponytail. He looked out of place and was working under the hood of his weathered vehicle. As we drove closer he leaned away from his car and waved. I was about to ask him directions when he smiled broadly and said, "Wow, it's you." He was around my age. His eyes held a thousand stories. I liked him immediately. This was a kindred spirit.

James bears no resemblance to my image of a colon hydrotherapist. He has a Pete Seeger-esque sensibility and looks like a fellow who has never missed a Grateful Dead concert in his life. We joked around while walking to his office. James was very warm and gracious, telling me he was proud of me for what I did. I was uncomfortable with compliments, though, particularly about the film. In my mind all I did was monumentally fuck up and survive.

At the office I met Madeline, his wife and business partner. We warmly hugged and exchanged pleasantries. She said James was excited to be working on me, and I couldn't help but respond, "It never occurred to me to use colonics and excitement in the same sentence."

"We do much more than that," she explained. "We do deep tissue massage and energy work as well."

James and Madeline abruptly shifted the tone of our conversation from light pleasantries to serious observation. "Do you understand that you will make a difference in people's lives?" said James. "Have you any idea how you touch people and help them on their journey?"

His focused intensity disarmed me. I felt a rumble of emotions in my solar plexus. What James said to me had collided with my deeply rooted belief in my unworthiness. How could I be so arrogant to think that what I had to say would make a difference in anyone else's life?

"I want to feel like I matter, but I just don't?" A heavy sadness pressed hard on my shoulders.

James knelt down beside my chair and looked me straight in the eyes. "Really hear me and feel what I say. This right now, this is who you are! You're not broken anymore, man."

James said that joy lay buried in a room deep in my heart, behind a door with rusty hinges. People like James and Madeline oil the hinges. They don't replace anything. They expose ancient wounds to fresh air and clean light, allowing the body and soul to heal itself.

After forty-five minutes of therapeutic irrigation, James said we could stop or go deeper. I thought he was referring to a deeper cleaning. He then began to delve into my abdomen, and it felt like he was reaching the core of my solar plexus.

As I relaxed into the process, my mind flashed with rapid-fire images. The past filled my brain. I saw the nuns, priests, and my father. I felt fear, emptiness, terror, betrayal, abandonment, and rage. It was as if the galactically overwhelming feelings of my past were condensed to a marble. I was breathing rapidly and perspiring. James asked me if I was okay, and I told him what was happening. I told him to continue. After the session we talked while he prepared his office for the morning. It was more like a debriefing than a dialogue.

As I got dressed I felt like I was straddling two dimensions. For a moment, there was no life or death, only creation. We breathe in and exhale. We ingest and expel. We expire and resume the cycle. No beginning—no end. All we can hold on to is illusion. Everything else is either unmanageable or out of our grasp. James and Madeline afforded me a glimpse into my inner light. James helped me on my quest toward awakening. We were like two pilgrims, one blind, the other lame. Alone, the journey is impossible. Together, the sighted lame man carried by the robust blind man reach their destination. In addition, they have the added benefit of forming a lifelong bond. I would never have arrived this far in life without the help of countless angels. In case you try to spot them, know that they rarely appear as you would imagine.

My initial approach to the spiritual path was linked to a healthy, or unhealthy, degree of skepticism. That day in the company of these fine radiant souls I knew I was a part of something bigger than myself. It was a lot to take in. I wasn't sure about how this applied to my life. All I knew was that everything felt right.

Later that afternoon Gregg and I drove to downtown Boulder to meet our hostess, Katrina, at a place called The Lazy Dog. Our table was outside overlooking a water playground. The play area was about 30 feet by 50 feet, and buried in the concrete rectangle were little holes that spritzed streams of water 6 feet high. It was like a hundred buried water pistols randomly going off. The time and location of where and when the water shot up was random. It was a vision of beautiful chaos. If the kids got wet, they laughed and cheered. If they guessed wrong, they still laughed. If you closed your eyes, you could hear and feel the joy. The sky was blue, the sun was warm, and the air was alive with the music of joyful children. All was right with the world. As I turned my attention back to my friends, Katrina's face held a somber, contemplative shadow.

"I'm jealous of those kids," said Katrina.

"Why is that?" I asked.

"Because I always had to be the adult in my house. My mother got really sick when I was two years old. After that, my dad just checked out. He was never emotionally present. From the time I was little, I had to take care of my siblings, my mom, and even my dad. I never got to do what those kids are doing."

I took her by the hand and led her to the middle of the fountain where all the kids watched us and giggled. We stood in one spot until the water started spouting, and we got wet. Katrina threw her head back and laughed with abandon, finding absolute joy in the spontaneity of that moment. In no time she was laughing harder than the children.

People will tell you what they need if you just listen closely. I was reminded that joy comes from the act of giving. In self-forgetting, I found peace and so did Katrina. I was serving my purpose.

After every screening of the documentary we invite the audience to ask questions. Some of the questions are funny. I was once asked to turn around because a woman wanted to see my backside. I asked her what she would think if a guy asked a woman in my position to do the same. The audience giggled nervously. I, of course, acquiesced and did my best *Project Runway* pirouette to high-pitched hoots and whistles.

Another woman asked, "Since you lost so much weight, do you, like, have, like, folds of skin hanging from your stomach and, like, if you do, would you consider, like, having them surgically removed?" This was asked in front of 160 people. I would not have the intestinal fortitude to ask such a question privately much less in front of a crowd. However, I didn't flinch and answered, "No, I do not."

People at these events privately reveal deeply personal information. After one screening a twenty-year-old woman approached me, looked into my eyes, and began weeping. I took her hand, and she continued to silently weep. When she stopped crying, I embraced her. She whispered, "Thank you." For a moment we took the same breaths and held each other in wordless compassion. She walked away never telling me the meaning of her tears. Sometimes the pain is too big for words. The most important thing to do is to hold a safe space for someone to express sadness.

At another screening a young woman came up to me with tears in her eyes and began speaking to me in Italian. She said her father was Sicilian. He had died a few months earlier, and she missed him. She said I reminded her of her father. She spoke about how she missed his warmth and affection and asked me to hold her for a moment. Then both of us wept, her for a father who had just passed away, me for the father I'd wished I'd had. I told her she was a beautiful human being. She looked at me and said, "I wish my father had told me that." I don't know why, but I replied, "Your father is talking to you right now. That was your father talking through me." She wept even harder and thanked me.

Apparently, I remind a lot of people of their father. I was awakened to how so many of us carry the same spiritual aches and pains.

When I listen to questions at these events, I see so many people yearning for compassion and intelligent guidance. This used to be the role of elders in various cultures. Their status was so auspicious that people lied about their age, claiming to be older to gain more respect. Our culture in the United States and many Western nations is just the opposite—people lie to appear younger, thinking that will make them more desirable.

A six-year-old girl in Des Moines sat in the front row with her mother and was the first person to raise her hand after the screening.

"Do you still talk to your daughter?" she asked.

"Yes, I do," I replied.

"Oh, good, good." She seemed very relieved and pleased by my answer.

I later learned her father was serving time for murder. She was really asking whether she would ever be able to talk to her father again. This little girl stayed next to me all evening as I spoke to people. I stumbled into a position where people offer me the most precious thing in the world: opening themselves up and giving me a glimpse into their heart.

A young woman from Eastern Europe wrote me after being diagnosed with multiple sclerosis. Her family didn't understand her condition and weren't supportive of her holistic approach to the illness. Because of the film, she felt inspired to find ways to feel more grateful and less despondent about her condition.

People don't always share their stories to receive an answer; they want to be heard. I don't know why or how the Universe saw fit to cross my path with these wonderful people. I just know that, when these people open their hearts, I see that love is everything. During these precious moments I forget myself and feel the magnificent reality that can only be experienced with an open heart.

I am in awe when I step on that stage and people applaud me for having corrected the mistakes in my life—a life characterized by a long trail of terrible decisions made at the worst possible times. I have no credentials other than a driver's license and a bachelor's degree in history. I haven't accomplished any noteworthy achievements, nor do I have any property or assets. I was an alcoholic and a drug addict who has recovered from a seemingly hopeless state. Yet, I find myself in front of hundreds of people who ask me questions about how to improve their lives.

We've had over a hundred showings of the documentary—Salt Lake City; Kansas City; Des Moines; Los Angeles; Washington, DC; Greenville, NC; Montclair, NJ; Seattle; Victoria, BC; Boulder; Martha's Vineyard, Boston. Crowds have ranged from five people in the back of a health food store to 1,200 at Agape International Spiritual Center, Los Angeles. Produced by Mikki Willis of Elevate and hosted by Michael Bernard Beckwith, it's shown in movie theaters, gymnasiums, school auditoriums, office conference rooms, and school classrooms. I've done Skype interviews with media outlets in Australia, Russia, and Singapore. I did a screening of the documentary and lecture at The Healthy Living Show and Aio Wira Spiritual Retreat both in Auckland, New Zealand. I kept asking myself, "How did I get here?"

I often worry about saying the right thing to a vulnerable person. People who love me tell me to just be myself, that I am right where I'm supposed to be. Nevertheless, I often feel inadequate to the task, as if the Universe has me confused with someone else. But the Universe is never confused. I, on the other hand, am very familiar with confusion. I am grateful to be alive and to have been given such an extraordinary opportunity to connect with so many people. I hope I am and will remain worthy of this gift.

No Platitudes in Prison

In 2010 there was a screening in a prison in Santa Rosa, north of San Francisco, before an audience of forty women, ranging in age from eighteen to sixty. These women were involved in a program called Starting Point designed to prevent recidivism.

I kept mulling over what I could say to these women after the screening that would possibly make a difference in their lives. New Age platitudes certainly wouldn't cut it here. I thought of my daughter, who was the same age as many of the inmates. Lisa was my first born, Daddy's little girl. What about these women in jail? Were they ever Daddy's little girl? Some must have been. In some cases, that may have been a bad thing. How did they end up in this place under such sad circumstances? Drug and alcohol abuse played a major role. So did abusive men.

We met in a large square room resembling a community college classroom. The inmates wore blue prison clothes similar to scrubs and sat in a circle accompanied by three prison staffers. Years of brutality and suffering had etched lines of sadness into their faces. I felt both discomfort and a wave of compassion as they turned their gazes on me, sizing up this male newcomer being sold to them as a spokesman for transformation. The women clapped after my host, Debbie Young, introduced me.

"Hi, everybody, my name is Frank, and I'm an alcoholic and an addict," I told them.

"Hi, Frank," they all chimed in. The event suddenly took on the atmosphere of a 12 Step meeting, affording me a bit of ease. But this was no church basement. This was jail. We were told before the talk that a twenty-two-year-old inmate had committed suicide the day before.

I shared stories about my boyhood, my fears, the violence at home and on the street. I talked about spiritual violence from the nuns and priests. I reflected on my cynicism, drug use, and the madness of it all. I spoke of my regrets, my hopes, my dreams. There were no platitudes. It was all real and from the heart.

The group was particularly interested in how I dealt with relapse. How do I get through the day when my mind is my enemy and all the snakes are out of the basket? I am no silver spoon kid with a bunch of answers. I see the ugliness in the world, and inside of myself, but the art of being human is appreciating the beauty in and around you in spite of the darkness. Life can be messy, ugly, and painful. It's like birth itself. There can be great joy in starting over, but many people are never afforded that privilege.

Throughout the meeting I noticed one woman with a frozen expression of sadness. Her face had not changed for an hour. When the time came for questions, the group went from gallows humor to stories of horrific abuse. Our time almost up, I looked at the women with the frozen gaze and asked her how she was doing. She paused and then replied, "I have never felt good about myself. I have voices in my head that are always beating me up."

Without thinking I got up and moved my chair and sat directly in front of her, our knees almost touching. We locked eyes, and I asked for her name.

"Nice to meet you, Mary," I said. "Do you feel safe?"

She hesitantly nodded. "Yes."

"Would you be willing to try something with me?"

She nodded and said, "Okay."

"Repeat after me. I am beautiful. I am sensual. I am intelligent. And I am worthy of love." At first she hesitated. A few women in the group spoke up with words of encouragement.

"I am beautiful," said Mary slowly, measuring her words. "I am sensual. I am intelligent. And I am worthy of love."

We repeated the affirmations together three times as she made eye contact with everyone in the circle. By the time Mary was done, her face had softened. The frozen expression of sadness melted. She actually started joking and giggling with the other inmates. A burden had been lifted, even if only temporarily.

It was one of the most gratifying experiences of my life. For a few brief minutes this woman had silenced the mean internal voices. She got a glimpse, a taste, maybe for the first time in a long time, maybe for the first time ever, of hope and possibilities. She opened up with me and allowed herself to be vulnerable because she sensed that I was just like her; I had been haunted by many of the same voices, and we both knew it. This was only one moment, not a cure. Only a glimpse into a possibility—there is always more work to be done.

Rekindling Hope

My story is for self-help devotees *and* for people who can't stand self-help—but desperately need it. It's also a socio-cultural romp through the New Age and wellness movements. Most of all, it's a journey about hope.

I am a flawed man. As I head out into glorious urban traffic, I just may flip you off. That doesn't diminish the work I've done or the desire to be a better person. I have transformed my life and found redemption in the midst of personal wreckage. The elements of my life that once shamed me are now a calling card that invites intimate conversations about forgiveness, love, redemption, emotional pain, and personal growth.

In less than four years, I went from being rescued in a grimy motel in Alameda to traveling the world speaking about transformation. My greatest flaws have become my greatest assets. Not even Frank Capra could have imagined a redemptive story like that.

At times I still take things personally, in contradiction to the second of the Four Agreements from the book with that title. The difference now is that I realize it sooner. The extent to which I take things personally is in direct proportion to how I'm taking care of myself. If I'm meditating, exercising, eating properly, and hanging out with positive people, I am better able to interpret what's going on around me as independent from myself.

I have learned that the three important things a man can say are: *I don't know. Would you please help me? I love you.* Not necessarily in that order.

Dealing with the causes and conditions of my obesity—my drug addictions and invisible demons—is a process. I had to head inward to the heart of addiction and despair, what Joseph Campbell calls the Hero's Journey. There is no secret to serious and sustained weight loss. Everyone knows the health benefits of exercise, fresh fruit and vegetables, and staying away from carbs and sugar. It's not rocket science. The challenging part— but by far the most rewarding and enduring part—is the emotional housecleaning.

A New Chapter

When I finally stopped feeling victimized, I understood the harsh reality that was my father's life. He was ten years old when his mother died. His father joined her four years later. At fourteen he was left to fend for himself in the madness of war-torn Europe. He was not loved, and so could not properly love me. My love for the three young men and their love for me was part of my healing journey. Three generations, one long past, all connected in a circle of love. And so it goes.

Whether you get your inspiration from Buddhism or Marianne Williamson, from ancient Judeo-Christian traditions or from psychedelics, all sources of metaphysical wisdom are connected by a common theme that centers on the power of love.

At times I feel like an imposter when I speak about the mind, body, spirit connection to wellness because there are aspects of my life in disarray. I console myself with the thought that I haven't pretended to be what I'm not. I am not an imposter. I am not lying to anybody. I only share my experiences and world view.

I wanted to be a teacher. In my heart of hearts teaching was always what I wanted to do. I went to college to challenge the belief that I was stupid. It never occurred to me that I would become a teacher in other ways. The world is a classroom, and at any given time I am either a student or a teacher. To be a teacher means to inspire and be inspired. The most important thing a teacher can do is to send a pupil home feeling better about him- or herself. Learning is an expression of life's purpose, alongside love. I consider teaching to be the highest form of optimism.

Ralph Waldo Emerson once said the measure of a man's success is how much he inspires the affection of his children and the respect of intelligent people. The commonality of the human experience became evident as I toured the country with the film. Wherever I went, people shared their process. They either had a desire to transform their lives or were in the midst of a transformation. The people I met welcomed the opportunity to share their experience. I believe that a common language invites community, and that language is the language of the heart.

I discovered that men have a yearning to change their lives but haven't found a corresponding language or permission to facilitate the shift they desire. The reality is that everyone in this life is on a spiritual journey. We're all on different routes and schedules. All anybody wants is a loving heart and peace of mind.

10

What the Journey Taught Me

Transformation is not for the faint of heart.

When things are out of sync in my life, I pause, get quiet, and breathe. That's my aspiration. Sometimes I get pissed and let the people around me know it! If that doesn't work, I ask for help. A broken mind, like a broken heart, cannot heal itself. That has been difficult for me to admit. Fears don't end; the way I face them does.

For most of my life I was filled with self-loathing and self-contempt. If anybody said to me what I said to myself, I'd have killed them. Since touring with the documentary, my life has been flooded with notes from thousands of loving people. I had to learn how to receive love. I'm still amazed that people want to hear what I have to say. I finally had to look at all of the emails and Facebook postings and admit to myself, "They can't all be wrong. I'm not smart enough to fool these many people."

Years have passed since my six-week adventure with the three amigos. I have recovered from acute withdrawal of narcotics, lost 120 pounds, worked through the anguish of heartbreak, and embraced a message of personal transformation. Today I weigh 185 pounds with a blood pressure of 100 over 70; there is no trace of hepatitis C; I eat a plant-based diet; my relationships with Mia and Lisa are healed; and I spend time with loving people. I work out frequently and try to keep my heart open now that I've learned it won't kill me if it's bruised. I've made many new friends and finally decided that maybe I have more value than I ever imagined.

Forgiveness opened my heart and nurtured my soul. Healthy food was one component. You can't just focus on the raw foods and veganism to explain what happened with me. It was an organic and harmonious collection of practices—and trial and error—that enabled me to become healthy and stay that way.

The older I get the more I realize how much I don't know. I was sure that by the time I reached this point in my life, I'd have more answers than questions. I was wrong. Fear ruled my life, so consequently I asked the wrong questions. I may not have received the answers I needed, but I got the answers I was comfortable with. One of my biggest discoveries was the only thing wrong with my life was my perception of it. Today I try to live with an undefended heart.

I have always indulged self-doubt rather than challenging it. I dealt with it by self-medicating with drugs, women, or money. As I mitigate the behaviors, I am left with myself. Fears and insecurities haven't gone away, but I face them from a different place. They no longer prevent me from fully experiencing the joys of living. I am no longer the frightened boy in a man's body waiting for the next beating from life. Anxiety and depression still creep in, but the spells are shorter and less frequent.

My experiences on the dark side are now my greatest assets. When I share my experience, a part of me heals. Do something nice for someone every day . . . and don't get caught.

I signed on to this journey with no knowledge of the destination. I discovered that all journeys have secret destinations of which the traveler remains unaware, even though ultimately we all end up in the same place. The journey continues.

"A good traveler has no fixed plans."—Lao Tzu.

Appendix

Resources for Your Own Transformation Journey

Food Matters

James and Laurentine are the dynamic duo behind the best-selling documentary films *Food Matters* and *Hungry for Change*. Graciously, they interviewed me for their film, *Hungry For Change*, and since we've become close friends. You can learn about their work and latest projects at FoodMatters.tv.

Your Wellness Connection

Dr. Michelle Robin is the founder of one of the nation's most successful integrative healing centers focusing on chiropractic, Chinese medicine, massage therapy, energy medicine, counseling, nutritional and wellness coaching, and movement arts.

7410 Switzer Road
Shawnee Mission, KS 66203
Toll Free: (877) 499-9355 (WELL)
yourwellnessconnection.com

"At Your Wellness Connection we meet people where they are, at their phase of health. We recognize that we are all on a journey toward wellness. No matter where someone lies on the continuum of health, we believe anyone can achieve their personal level of wellness" (www.yourwellness connection.com/about-us/our-philosophy).

Cleanse Easy

cleanseasy@gmail.com
CleanseEasy.com

Shayla Mihaly will support you as you learn how easy cleansing can be— and should be! Cleanse Easy is an easy cleansing and weight-loss system that works with great success. The Cleanse Easy program is designed to go anywhere. You can cleanse, detox and lose weight— without interrupting your daily schedule. If you work long hours, have kids, and/or travel a lot, you can still do this cleanse successfully! It's easy, affordable, powerful, and can easily fit into your daily life, right now.

Raven Crystals

432 N Ventura Ave
Ventura, CA 93001
RavenCrystals.com

Raven Crystals carries amazing crystals, mineral specimens, and hand-crafted crystal products from around the world. Raven Crystals also provides information about the care, metaphysical properties, and healing attributes of crystals, mineral specimens, and stones. The crystals found at Raven Crystals are hand selected based on their beauty, healing attributes, uniqueness, and collectible qualities. Every crystal order is gathered, wrapped, and packaged with loving care and intention. The proprietor of Raven Crystals, Andrea Lehr, is an artist, Reiki master, energy worker, shaman, and massage practitioner for animals and people.

Peace Yoga Gallery

903 South Main Street
Los Angeles, CA 90015
Phone: (213) 500-5007
peaceyogagallery.com

Cheri Rae, owner: "Stuck in traffic? Can't find parking? Late? Breathe . . . slow down. There is no 'late' at Peace Yoga. You will arrive exactly when you are supposed to and we will welcome you."

Rejuvenation and Performance Institute at Grace Grove

PO Box 4195
Sedona, AZ 86340
Email: team@rpinstitute.com
Phone: (928) 649-0456
Fax: (888) 820-4158

"Rejuvenation and Performance Institute (RPI) is a state-of-the-art life crisis and total wellness management firm. Focused on assisting clients to reach Peak Performance, RPI offers solutions-centered advisory and consulting programs for the world's top-level executives and their support teams. Based at the Grace Grove Lifestyle Center in Sedona, Arizona, RPI is set amidst a 25-acre campus in forested nature. Secluded and surrounded by the ever-running waters of Oak Creek, Grace Grove openly receives time-stressed CEO's, C-Level executives, and collaborative executive teams.

"All of our programs and offerings support digestive healing, proper immune function and physical, mental, and spiritual wellness. . . . Our main goal is to move people safely and gracefully toward a state of optimum health and peak performance" (www.rpinstitute.com/about-grace -grove/).

The Hoffman Process

Phone: (800) 502-5353

"Founded in 1967, the Hoffman Process is a week-long residential and personal-growth retreat that helps participants identify negative behaviors, moods and ways of thinking that developed unconsciously and were conditioned in childhood.

"The Process will help you become conscious of and disconnect from negative patterns of thought and behaviors on an emotional, intellectual, physical and spiritual level in order to make significant positive changes in your life. You will learn to remove habitual ways of thinking and behaving, align with your authentic self, and respond to situations in your life from a place of conscious choice" (www.hoffmaninstitute.org/the-hoffman -process/). *The Hoffman Process is conducted thirty times a year in the United States.*

Getting Your Wheatgrass

Keep in mind that as a nutrient-dense food, wheatgrass juice consumption can cause your body to detox, and this detoxification can, in turn, produce temporary side effects such as nausea and diarrhea. That's what happened to me. But don't let these temporary symptoms of detox dissuade you from trying one of nature's most potent healthy foods.

Fresh wheatgrass is sold in health food stores and in vegan or vegetarian restaurants. Some Asian markets also carry wheatgrass. Some of you may want to grow and then juice wheatgrass yourself to ensure a constant and high-quality supply. Here are some resources you can draw upon:

- How to Grow Wheatgrass at Home (www.wikihow.com/Grow -wheatgrass-at-Home) is a useful website which will take you through the steps.

- Go to YouTube and check out videos listed under the search string "How to Grow Wheatgrass."
- On Amazon.com you will find certified organic wheatgrass growing kits.
- At Sproutpeople.org you can purchase wheatgrass seeds and grow kits.
- Also at wheatgrass.org find wheatgrass kits and seeds.
- At vitaminshoppe.com you have access to wheatgrass powder and wheatgrass tablets if you choose to bypass growing it yourself. The powder has a longer shelf life than un-juiced wheatgrass and can be mixed with other drinks.

Finding Raw Foods and Vegan Restaurants

When traveling, especially in other countries, you may find it a challenge to identify raw foods and vegan restaurants. Fortunately, there are some resources which will help you in your healthy fine dining quest.

- The website happycow.net has a search engine to find good raw foods, vegan, or vegetarian restaurants just about anywhere on the planet, whether you are in Serbia or Russia or Turkey or Argentina or any points in between. Did you know, for instance, that Germany has more than 1,200 such restaurants? Italy has nearly 800, and Thailand nearly 500. You will find at least 11,000 such restaurants in the United States, from nineteen in North Dakota to more than 2,000 in California.
- If you are a connoisseur of healthy fine dining and prefer only the best, you might check out www.foodandwine.com/slide-shows/best-vegan-and-vegetarian-restaurants. There you will find what are considered by culinary experts to be the twenty best gourmet raw foods, vegan, and vegetarian restaurants in the United States from Kajitsu in New York City, to Vedge in Philadelphia, Elizabeth's Gone Raw in Washington, DC,

Green Seed Vegan in Houston, Café Gratitude in Venice, CA, and Greens in San Francisco.

The Most Popular Raw Foods Retreats in the United States

While these retreats may seem designed primarily for people with health issues, anyone can derive some seriously good health benefits from attending a week or more of the sessions offered by these raw foods health spas. These retreats provide a ready-made support group, much like I experienced with the three amigos, to assist you in making healthy lifestyle choices and transforming your life for the better.

Two retreats stand out for offering a wide variety of health services other than just wheatgrass and raw foods—yoga, massage, colonics, far-infrared saunas, blood work analysis, educational health counseling, and much more. (You can also access a raw foods retreat directory, listed by country, at www.retreatfinder.com/directory/food/raw_food.aspx.)

- Epic Living Retreats. Amber Zuckswert, founder: "Escape the grind for an unforgettable wellness adventure. Balance, unite, and invigorate your mind, body, and spirit in paradise with a 7–10 day all-inclusive retreat or training intensive featuring international renowned experts. We teach you the skills you'll need for radiant health and longevity. Then help you integrate and design them into your lifestyle. Costa Rican culture and stunning natural environment set the stage for our adventures" (epiclivingretreats.com and epicself.com).
- Hippocrates Health Institute. Probably the oldest raw foods health spa in the nation, if not the world, is located in West Palm Beach, Florida. Codirectors (and husband and wife team) Dr. Brian Clement and Dr. Anna Maria Clement have published many books about the benefits of their program to transform human health. Tens of thousands of people worldwide have attended their one-, two-, and three-week programs. They also offer an intensive nine-week program

for people who want to become health educators utilizing the Hippocrates prescription for regaining and maintaining good health. Find out more atHippocratesinstitute.org.

- Tree of Life Center. Located in Patagonia, Arizona, and founded in the early 1990s by Dr. Gabriel Cousens, this retreat offers detoxification sessions and green juice fasting along with a holistic array of other health services. Spiritual nutrition programs are also offered. Dr. Cousens has authored several books setting forth the health rejuvenation ideas on which his retreat operates. One of his health specialties is treating diabetes using holistic practices. Find out more attreeoflife.nu.

Finding a Somatic Practitioner

Releasing traumas and accumulated emotional baggage held in your body, as I experienced with a massage therapist, may require a practitioner trained in some form of somatic bodywork. Peter A. Levine, PhD, a pioneer in this field, maintains the Somatic Experiencing Trauma Institute in Boulder, Colorado, which has a three-year training program for people to use somatic bodywork as a therapeutic practice. The Institute has a practitioner directory available to search at www.traumahealing .com/somatic-experiencing/practitioner-directory.html.

There are also somatic practitioner registries for other countries. For example, in Britain you will find a Somatic Experiencing Association listing atseauk.org.uk.

Finding a Colonics Practitioner

Otherwise known as colon hydrotherapy, if you want to get a colonics treatment as I did to help with your detoxification process, you can find several national and international registries of certified practitioners. There is the International Association and Register of Integrative Colon Therapists and Trainers at colonic-association.net. You might also try the International Association for Colon Hydrotherapy located at www.healthy.net/Alternative_Health/Association/IACT_International _Association_for_Colon_Hydrotherapy/17.

Both of these groups and their websites will not only give you lists of colon hydrotherapists in your area, but also provide lots of good information about the colonics process itself, what you can expect from it, and answers to some of the more commonly asked questions about the procedure. You may be surprised at how many practitioners are around you. If you search in Texas, for instance, you will find twenty-one different cities, from large metropolises like Dallas and Houston to small towns like Tyler, spread across the state with certified colon hydrotherapists listed in the registry.

Advanced Colonic Techniques Clinic

JamesAllred.com/colonhydrotherapy

James Allred began practicing colon hydrotherapy in 1977. In his Boulder clinic James facilitates unprecedented sessions based in the mechanics and functions of the soma. James also provides practical training and mentoring for students by and through experience making each opportunity unique.

Fluid Water Therapy

Fluid Water Therapy
22 East 21st Street
Suite 6R
New York, NY 10010
Phone: (212) 888-9116
fluidwatertherapy.com

Fluid Water Therapy is a colon hydrotherapy clinic in Manhattan that provides state-of-the-art intestinal detoxification and wellness guidance in an intimate and comfortable environment. Fluid utilizes the FDA-registered

Angel of Water colon hydrotherapy system to provide maximum comfort, hygiene, and intestinal waste removal. The treatment water undergoes a comprehensive bacterial-eradication process including six stages of filtration, double-UV light processing, and ozone sanitization. The clinic's services are particularly effective for those who are struggling with weight loss, body detoxification, and chronic conditions. In full compliance with HIPAA guidelines, all patients can rest assured that their sessions are fully confidential.

Fluid is owned and operated by Dr. Francis Gonzalez, ND, an I-ACT certified colon hydrotherapist and instructor, with over ten years of experience managing colon hydrotherapy clinics in New York, Maryland, and the Caribbean.

References

Adzersen, Karl-Heinrich, P. Jess, K. W. Freivogel, I. Gerhard, and Gunther Bastert. 2003. "Raw and Cooked Vegetables, Fruits, Selected Micronutrients, and Breast Cancer Risk: A Case-Control Study in Germany." *Nutrition and Cancer* 46(2): 131–137.

Agren, Jyrki, J., E. Tvrzicka, Mikko T. Nenonen, T. Helve, and Osmo Hänninen. 2001. "Divergent Changes in Serum Sterols during a Strict Uncooked Vegan Diet in Patients with Rheumatoid Arthritis." *British Journal of Nutrition* 85(2): 137–139.

Carson, James W., Francis J. Keefe, Veeraindar Goli, Ann Marie Fras, Thomas R. Lynch, Steven R. Thorp, and Jennifer L. Buechler. 2005. "Forgiveness and Chronic Low Back Pain: A Preliminary Study Examining the Relationship of Forgiveness to Pain, Anger, and Psychological Distress." *The Journal of Pain* 6(2): 84–91.

Chodron, Pema. 2012. *Living Beautifully with Uncertainty and Change*. Boston: Shambhala Publications, Inc.

Cox, Susie S., Rebecca J. Bennett, Thomas M. Tripp, and Karl Aquino. 2012. "An Empirical Test of Forgiveness Motives' Effects on Employees' Health and Well-being." *Journal of Occupational Health Psychology* 17(3): 330–340.

De Stefani, Eduardo, Paolo Boffetta, Alvaro L. Ronco, Pelayo Correa, Fernando Oreggia, Hugo Deneo-Pellegrini, Maria Mendilaharsu, and Juan Leiva.

2005. "Dietary Patterns and Risk of Cancer of the Oral Cavity and Pharynx in Uruguay." *Nutrition and Cancer* 51(2): 132–139.

Emmons, Robert A., and Robin Stern. 2013. "Gratitude as a Psychotherapeutic Intervention." *Journal of Clinical Psychology* 69(8): 846–855.

Forgive For Good. 2014. Accessed July 29. http://learningtoforgive.com.

Greater Good: The Science of a Meaningful Life. 2014. "What Is Gratitude?" Accessed September 17. http://greatergood.berkeley.edu/topic/gratitude /definition.

Larsen, Britta A., Ryan S. Darby, Christine R. Harris, Dana K. Nelkin, Per-Erik Milam, and Nicholas J. Christenfeld. 2012. "The Immediate and Delayed Cardiovascular Benefits of Forgiving." *Psychosomatic Medicine* 74(7): 745–750.

Lawler-Row, Kathleen A., Johan C. Karremans, Cynthia Scott, Meirav Edlis-Matityahou, and Laura Edwards. 2008. "Forgiveness, Physiological Reactivity and Health: The Role of Anger." *International Journal of Psychophysiology* 68(1): 51–58.

Levi, Fabio, C. Pasche, Carlo La Vecchia, Francesca Lucchini, and Silvia Franceschi. 1999. "Food Groups and Colorectal Cancer Risk." *British Journal of Cancer* 79(7–8): 1283–1287.

Levine, Peter A. *Waking the Tiger: Healing Trauma*. 1997. Berkeley: North Atlantic Books.

Pellegrini, Nicoletta, Emma Chiavaro, Claudio Gardana, Teresa Mazzeo, Daniele Contino, Monica Gallo, Patrizia Riso, Vincenzo Fogliano, and Marisa Porrini. 2010. "Effect of Different Cooking Methods on Color, Phytochemical Concentration, and Antioxidant Capacity of Raw and Frozen Brassica Vegetables." *Journal of Agricultural and Food Chemistry* 58(7): 4310–4321.

Quote Investigator. 2012. "It's Easy to Quit Smoking. I've Done It a Thousand Times." Accessed July 29, 2014. http://quoteinvestigator.com/2012/09/19 /easy-quit-smoking/.

Schucman, Helen. 2007. *A Course in Miracles*. Mill Valley: Foundation for Inner Peace.

Svalina, Suncica S., and Jon R. Webb. 2012. "Forgiveness and Health among People in Outpatient Physical Therapy." *Disability and Rehabilitation* 34(5): 383–392.

Tang, Li, Gary R. Zirpoli, Khurshid Guru, Kirsten B. Moysich, Yuesheng Zhang, Christine B. Ambrosone, and Susan E. McCann. 2010. "Intake of

References

Cruciferous Vegetables Modifies Bladder Cancer Survival." *Cancer Epidemiology, Biomarkers & Prevention* 19(7): 1806–1811.

Williamson, Marianne. 2010. *A Course in Weight Loss: 21 Spiritual Lessons for Surrendering Your Weight Forever.* Hay House.

Acknowledgments

How do you describe the indescribable? Cat Maida entered my life four years ago. We met at a screening in Kansas City. We didn't just look at each other, we saw each other. There was a deeper knowing at play. Something beyond my narrow vision. My heart was ahead of my brain. Thank God for that. When I had surgery, she slept in the hospital for a week. It was Christmas. She bought a little tree and bars of chocolates for the nurses. For the next six months she nursed me back to health. During the year of my recovery I was barely able to walk. She was there. Her love for me was unwavering. It was a love beyond my comprehension. It was deep, it was pure, it was real. At times I was at a loss. I didn't know how to receive such a heart. Cat shows me what love looks like every day. Sometimes I am afraid of how much I love her. I am in awe of her courageous heart.

I loved her yesterday. I love her now. I will love her forever.

Cat loved me in spite of my fears and insecurities. To my amazement, she always saw past my flaws. I never knew a love like this. She is my light in the storm; she is the echo of my heartbeat. Sometimes I feel like she has always been there in spirit waiting for my body to arrive.

I have not been an easy person to be with. I can be moody and dark.

But Cat always sees the light.

The thought of her out of my life is unbearable. It is the price of love.

Cat has opened my heart and mind to love. Her actions defy my fear-based barriers.

Thank you, Cat, for tirelessly typing and retyping the manuscript. For seeing in me what I could not or would not see in myself. If I designed my perfect lover, she would never have measured up to you.

I never thought I'd ever get to do this. Miracles do happen! There are people whom I would like to acknowledge for being a part of my life.

To my mother and father, thank you for giving me life.

To Izzy, the best brother in the world, for your steadfast love and encouragement and my infinitely patient sister-in-law Kat.

My sister, Saint Rosalie, for your unwavering loving spirit. I love you Roe!

Vinnie Modica for loving me through my heroin addiction.

To Jeff Lamont, artistic genius and brother from another mother who supported me in every way.

To Gregg Marks, for your spiritual wisdom, vision, and patience.

Ryland, Carey, and Conor for your dedication and love.

Dr. Joel Lopez, for your intelligent and compassionate practice in the art of medicine.

Shayla Mihaly, for introducing me to the joys of colonic irrigation.

Robert Keehan, for challenging my perceived limits and working out with me for over a year. I lost over a hundred pounds working out with Robert. We still haven't found them.

Richard Salles, crazy friend and lawyer.

Mike Federici, neighborhood gangster and confidant.

Marianne Williamson, whose influence inspired me to finish the book.

To Jason Mraz, for your music, your kindness, and your soul.

To Professor Lunine, who told me to relax and study Gandhi for two semesters.

Professor Saul Steier, chair of the humanities MA program, for admitting me.

Acknowledgments

Norman Penn, for being my older brother, introducing me to Lenny Bruce, Phillip Roth, Yiddish wisdom, and weed.

To Andrea Lehr, my friend and confidante. Thank you for sifting through volumes of transcripts.

Valerie Higgins, for your intuition and love—you took the time to check on me and saved my life. Thank you Ms. Higgins.

Michelle Robbin for your loyalty, support, friendship, and your passionate dedication to making a difference in people's lives every day.

The fabulous Crystal Jenkins and the amazing staff at the Hoffman Institute.

Carla Mandilli, MD, my dear friend and psychiatrist for guiding me through an eclipse.

Natalia and Sean Maida for being perfect, just like your Momma.

To my friends Morgan Langan, Puma St. Angel, Dennis Little, Dave Pappas, and Tony Paoli for believing in me.

Vinnie Biasi for showing me that a man can be gentle without sacrificing his masculinity.

Elaine Palmer, for those long talks off the ledge and back to reality.

Danny Kenny, for always blessing me before I leave his home.

Dale Sclafani, we're still standing, bro!

Debra Olliver, for helping me start it all.

Dr. Anita Gadhia Smith, we've come a hell of a long way.

Randall Fitzgerald, for all your work.

Jimmy Nesfield, thanks for being there.

Peter (Rocky) Braun for shelter at the "Inn."

It took a long time and a lot of people to get me to this point. I didn't mention everyone important to my journey. I had to save some for the next book.

Index

About the Author

F rank was born in Brooklyn, New York, on August 26, 1951. According to his astrological chart, "peace and harmony are my battle cry." The chart further claims that he is "flashy but not gaudy and prefers to dress elegantly." His sartorial preferences reflect a greater spiritual depth. Frank's resume is "eclectic." He has been, in no particular order, a NY City cab driver, scrap metal hauler, dishwasher, census taker, mail boy, ditch digger, bouncer, illegal narcotics distributor, general contractor, actor, radio announcer, carpenter, avid reader, seeker of God, weight gain/weight loss aficionado, recovered alcoholic/junkie, cocaine crazy, smoker, speed freak; raw foodist, vegan, BBQ connoisseur, lover, hater, father, husband, grad student, good guy, bad guy, social activist.

Frank is the subject of the award-winning documentary *May I Be Frank* and is featured in the documentary *Hungry For Change*. These films reflect Frank's journey back to health and spiritual redemption. Frank is an international spokesperson for personal transformation.

Frank does not claim to be an expert or have *the* answer. He has witnessed the indisputable fact that we are all connected. What we do can and will make a difference. Frank learned that the three most important things a man can say are: *I don't know. Would you please help me? I love you.*